Diary of a Deployed Doc

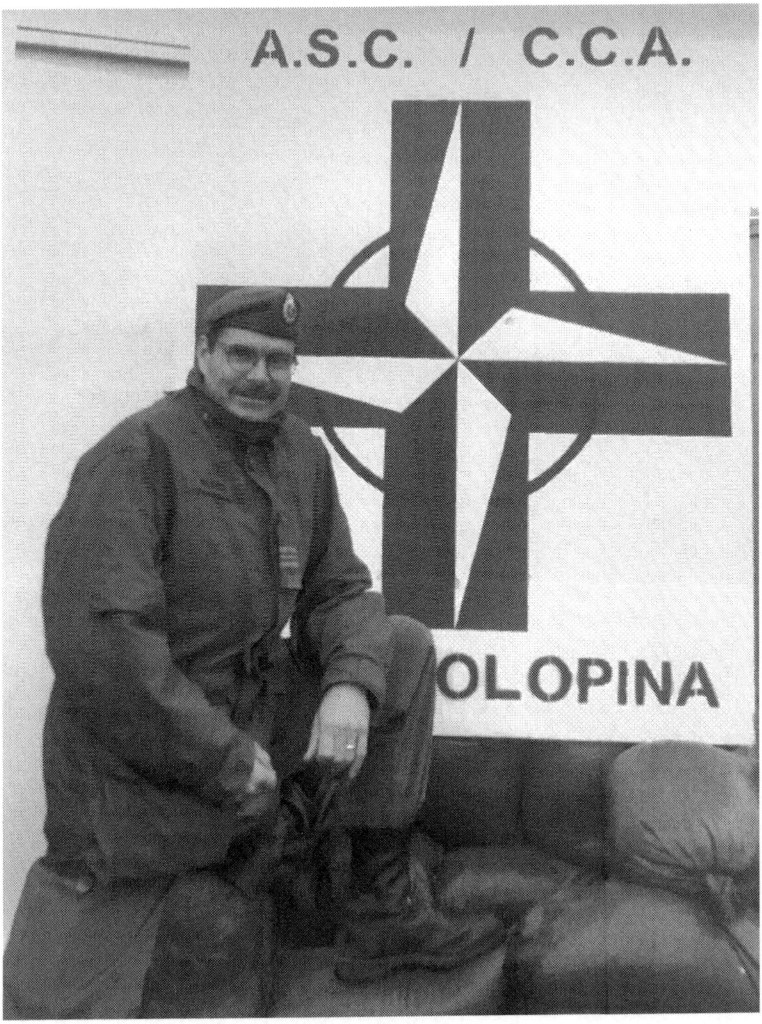

Major (Retired) Darrell Menard OMM, CD2, BPE, MA, MD, Dip Sport Med

ISBN 978-1-0689493-0-2

Cover design and illustrations by Rebecca Menard

Book design and production by Jennifer Pershick

Printed in Canada

Second Edition

Table of Contents

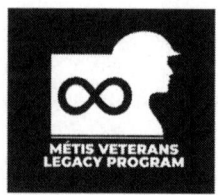

Acknowledgements

I wish to take this opportunity to thank the many people who played an important role in helping to get this book published. The Métis Veterans Legacy Program generously provided the funding for this project and its staff played a significant role in ensuring that this project successfully made it through all the hoops that needed to be jumped through. Indigenous artist Rebecca Menard, created all the artwork for this project. Matthew Menard is an Indigenous physician, and he was a huge help in editing my original manuscript. My wife, Janet, helped with editing but, more importantly, single-handedly supported our family throughout my deployment. I am very grateful to Patricia Walsh who meticulously edited this work in preparation for publishing. Master Warrant Officer Nancy Tsintsadze was very helpful in locating several retired military personnel who appear in the photographs in this book. Jennifer Pershick did the formatting for this book and played a key role in arranging for its publication. I would also like to thank all the Canadian Armed Forces personnel with whom I had the privilege to serve on this deployment and those who continue to put their lives on the line to make our world a safer place. Lastly, I would like to honour all the Indigenous people who have served in the Canadian Armed Forces, particularly those who have given their lives in the service of others. The views expressed in the book are those of the author and not those of the Department of National Defence or the Canadian Armed Forces. Megwetch!

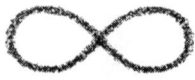

Abbreviations

Canadian Armed Forces personnel are often accused of speaking a unique language because of the number of acronyms they use for just about everything. I hope this index will make it easier for readers to better understand all the terms used in this book.

AAG – Arrival Assistance Group

ACLS – Advanced Cardiac Life Support

AOR – area of responsibility

ASC – Advanced Surgical Centre

AWACS – Airborne Warning and Control System

BG – Battle Group

BGen – Brigadier-General

ATLS – Advanced Trauma Life Support

CAF – Canadian Armed Forces

Capt – Captain

CCSFOR – Canadian Contingent Stabilization Force

CD2 – Canadian Forces' Decoration, 2nd Clasp

CDS – Chief of the Defence Staff

CF – Canadian Forces

CFB – Canadian Forces Base

CANEX – Canadian Forces Exchange System

CISM – Conseil international du sport militaire / International
        Military Sports Council

CO – Commanding Officer

Col – Colonel

COM Z HQ – Communications Zone Headquarters

Cpl – Corporal

CSM – Company Sergeant Major

CWO – Chief Warrant Officer

DAG – Departure Assistance Group

DART – Disaster Assistance Response Team

DCDS – Deputy Chief of the Defence Staff

DCO – Deputy Commanding Officer

DLO – Divisional Liaison Officer

DM – Deutsche Mark (exchange rate was DM x .927 = CAN$)

DND – Department of National Defence

DNZ – Democratic People's Union (Bosnia-Herzegovina)

DPRE – displaced persons, refugees, evacuees

ECG – electrocardiogram

EEG – electroencephalogram

ETA – estimated time of arrival

FART – Fast Action Response Team

G4 – Logistics Officer at Army Headquarters

HLVW – Heavy Logistic Vehicle Wheeled

HQ – headquarters

ICU – intensive care unit

IFOR – Implementation Force

ILS – imaginary lat syndrome

IRT – Immediate Response Team

ISO – International Organization for Standardization

IV – intravenous line

JAG – Judge Advocate General officer

J1 Med – Joint Staff Medical Officer

J Staff – Joint Staff

JTF – joint task force

LCol – Lieutenant-Colonel

LGen – Lieutenant-General

LS – Leading Seaman

MCpl – Master Corporal

Med A – medical assistant

MI – myocardial infarction

MIR – medical inspection room

MLVW – Medium Logistic Vehicle Wheeled

MND – Multi-National Division
MND/SW – Multi-National Division South-West
MO – medical officer
MP – military police
MRE – meals ready to eat
NATO – North Atlantic Treaty Organization
NCE – National Command Element
NCM – non-commissioned member
NCO – non-commissioned officer
NDHQ – National Defence Headquarters
NDMC – National Defence Medical Centre
NVG – night vision goggles
O Company – Oscar Company
O-Group – Orders Group
OMM – Order of Military Merit
OPP – Ontario Provincial Police
Op/ops – Operation/operations
OR – operating room
PER – Personnel Evaluation Report
PsychO – psychologist
PTSD – post-traumatic stress disorder
PX – Post Exchange
RCR – Royal Canadian Regiment
Recce – reconnaissance
REMF – rear echelon mother($#!+&*%)
RFP – Roto Four problem
Roto – rotation
RPG – rocket-propelled grenade
R&R – rest and recuperation
RSM – Regimental Sergeant Major
RTM – return to momma
SDA – Party of Democratic Action (Bosnia-Herzegovina)

SFOR – Stabilization Force

Sgt – Sergeant

SIV – staff inspection visit

STRATEVAC – strategic evacuation

TOW – tube-launched, optically-tracked, wire-guided missile

UMS – unit medical station

UN – United Nations

UNHCR – United Nations High Commissioner for Refugees

UNPROFOR – United Nations Protection Force

UXO – unexploded explosive ordnance

VK – Velika Kladusa (Bosnia-Herzegovina)

WO – Warrant Officer

WSE – while so employed

ZAP number – a personal identification number

Introduction

Many Indigenous people have made significant contributions to the success of the Canadian Armed Forces (CAF) during numerous wars and peacekeeping efforts all over the world. Literally thousands of First Nations, Inuit and Métis men and women have volunteered to serve a nation that has often treated them as second-class citizens. Despite this, they have served Canada loyally, and many of these brave ancestors even lost their lives fighting for freedoms they themselves did not enjoy back home. In recognition of their valuable contributions, many Canadian Indigenous war veterans have been awarded decorations for bravery. Tragically, many of these same veterans did not receive treatment equal to other Canadian war veterans when they returned to Canada. I am proud to be a Métis veteran and honoured to be in the company of these exceptional people.

I am Major (Retired) Darrell Menard, and my ancestors are from the Métis Nation Homeland (Manitoba). As a Canadian Forces physician I was fortunate to serve my country in the effort to bring peace and stability to Bosnia, a country devastated by war. Over my forty-year military career, I had the opportunity to serve my country in many different capacities, including as a paymaster, physical education and recreation officer, athlete, coach, author, peacekeeper, physician, educator, sport medicine specialist, and Indigenous person. As part of my employment with the Canadian Armed Forces, my family and I were posted to many different parts of Canada where we had the opportunity to make lifelong friendships and to enjoy the diverse beauty of our wonderful nation. The military also provided me with the opportunity to travel all over the world.

My career as an officer in the Canadian Armed Forces has had many highlights, one of which was my seven-month tour in war-torn Bosnia, where I served as the medical advisor to the Commanding Officer of the Canadian Contingent Stabilization Force (CCSFOR) from

July 1998 until February 1999. The following narrative is a day-to-day diary of my experiences, thoughts and feelings during my deployment in Bosnia. By sharing my personal story with you, I hope to offer you some insight into the life that Canadian military personnel experience while on deployment. Megwetch!

How It All Started

While my departure date for this deployment was set for the 12th of July 1998, the adventure truly began in early March 1998 when my boss first informed me that my name was being considered for the role of medical advisor to the Commanding Officer for CCSFOR in Bosnia. This happened immediately prior to my travelling to Ireland with the Canadian Armed Forces Running team competing in the Conseil international du sport militaire (CISM) World Military Cross-Country Championships. I was told I was fourth on the list of personnel being considered, but the chances of my being selected were minuscule. The morning I returned from Ireland, I was informed that I had managed to rise to second on the list, but the number one choice really wanted to go, and it was simply a matter of waiting for his formal acceptance. At the end of the same day, I was informed that I had become the "Chosen One," and I would be deploying with the third rotation of CAF personnel (Roto 3) in mid-July. When asked how I felt about this tasking, I answered that it wasn't something on my bucket list but that I would go if no one else was available. Not a very enthusiastic response, but it was truly how I felt at the time. I think many people were surprised that I didn't threaten to put in for my release from the military, but I have always viewed this kind of tactic as disloyal – if you honestly felt that way, it was time to seriously consider finding a new line of employment.

It took some time to get over the initial shock of being selected, and then I began to think of the enormous impact that a seven-month tour would have on my life and my family. I would not be there to support Janet during the final stages of her nurse practitioner training. Nor would I be there for Nathan's birthday, Janet's graduation, my medical class's tenth reunion, Matthew's first days at university, Christmas and New Year's. My private practice would come to a grinding halt, and all those folks who have come to depend on Janet and me for regular and after-hours medical care would have to be seen elsewhere. This would be painful both personally and financially. I would miss half my old timers' soccer season, and I would no longer be able to help coach my daughter Rebecca's soccer team. I would also need to complete extra medical and military training in the brief time before my departure. To add to my concerns, I had no idea who would look after my primary military responsibilities while I was away. If my boss brought someone in to replace me, would I still have my job when I returned? I should also mention that I was already feeling quite burnt-out from dealing with the demands of my military responsibilities, my moonlighting work caring for patients, my family's needs and the stress of competing as an endurance runner.

At one point, I took a moment to say the following prayer: "Lord, I am trying to be a good person, but I am really struggling to do all the things I have on my plate. I really need something to change, and I am asking for your help." Several days after saying this prayer, I found myself being considered for this deployment. You really do need to be careful what you pray for because God may intervene in ways that you don't fully understand at the time. As you can tell, I was focused on all the things that this deployment would take away from me. As things evolved, I began to try and focus on all the good that could come from being part of this deployment. I must admit that you begin to question what you are getting yourself into when everyone you meet asks you how you feel about having to go to Bosnia and then warns you to keep your head down and your feet on the hard top.

At this point, I think it would be worthwhile to explain why I was being deployed to Bosnia as part of a contingent of Canadian soldiers. In 1990, the Federal Republic of Yugoslavia collapsed, resulting in the displacement of over two million men, women and children. Unfortunately, this region disintegrated into a brutal "ethnically rooted" civil war that took the lives of approximately one hundred thousand people. The fighting that occurred in this region would most accurately be described as a campaign of war crimes that included ethnic cleansing and genocide. Much of the destruction that occurred during this period of horrific violence was focused on the region known as Bosnia-Herzegovina.

Hoping to put an end to the violence, the international community finally stepped in. From 1992 to 1995, Canada contributed troops to the United Nations Protection Force (UNPROFOR). This group was tasked with protecting non-combatants and establishing security in the region. This effort was a success, and in 1995 the North Atlantic Treaty Organization (NATO) imposed a final ceasefire known as the Dayton Peace Accords. To ensure that this delicate ceasefire was maintained, Canada was asked to contribute personnel to the Multinational Peace Implementation Force (IFOR). In 1996, this IFOR phase ended, and a Stabilization Force (SFOR) phase began. The SFOR phase lasted until 2010, and I deployed with the third rotation (Roto 3) of Canadians supporting this stabilization force.

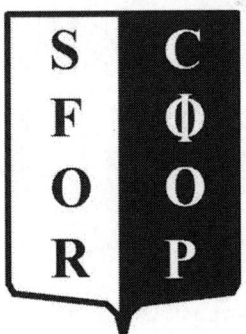

Over the years, approximately forty thousand Canadian Armed Forces personnel served in Bosnia on peace-supporting missions designed to protect the lives of civilians and to allow for stabilization and reconstruction initiatives. CAF personnel contributed to important work that included monitoring demining efforts, hunting down suspected war criminals, helping with weapons collection and destruction, monitoring and assisting with fair elections, rebuilding and repairing badly damaged infrastructure and offering humanitarian assistance. This contribution often required our military personnel to live in challenging conditions, spending many months away from their families – and it ultimately cost twenty-three Canadian Armed Forces personnel their lives. I hope that my diary account helps to highlight efforts by Canadian military personnel to help the people of Bosnia reconstruct their severely damaged country.

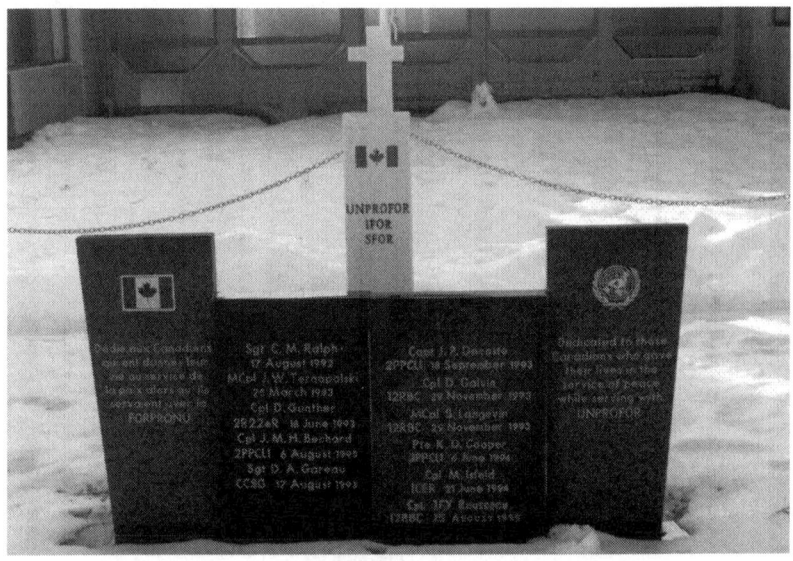

A cenotaph honouring some of the Canadian military personnel who gave their lives to establish peace in Bosnia.

The idea of going to the former Yugoslavia became a reality for me when I was given one-and-a-half-days' notice to be in Canadian Forces Base (CFB) Petawawa and begin fourteen days of pre-deployment training. In those thirty-six hours, I had to draw all my combat clothing and equipment, pick up all my administrative, dental and medical documents, undergo a full dental assessment, and find my dog tags, passport, security clearance, ID passes, and so on. To the credit of our military bureaucracy, when something is operationally required, you are moved straight to the front of the line. To my utter amazement, I completed nearly everything I was asked to do prior to reporting to Petawawa. At 0520hrs ("O dark thirty" in military time) on the 14th of April 1998, I jumped into my car and headed to CFB Petawawa in full combat clothing – feeling as out of place as a ballet dancer trying out for a professional football team. The combat uniform I was issued felt very foreign, and my combat boots weren't even slightly broken in. I made the trip in a rusty Honda Accord full of equipment that I had no idea how to wear or use, and as I drove through the front gates of the base, I realized how very "Army" the world I was entering truly was. Everyone and everything I saw was lean, mean and very green.

This was a huge change from my regular life at National Defence Medical Centre (NDMC), where I spend my days sitting in a sterile office making decisions regarding employment limitations for ill and injured military personnel. In my world, no one ever comes to work in a combat uniform, there are no armoured vehicles in the parking lot, and the closest thing to a weapon you can find in the building is a very dull letter opener. But as I arrived at the base, I realized that I was entering a world quite foreign to an older, operationally inexperienced, headquarters-based, Air Force medical officer and that I had very little time to learn a lot of things that would be very important to my survival in Bosnia. The feeling was not dissimilar to walking into my first class at medical school and realizing how much I didn't know and just how big a responsibility I was taking on. What I did have going for me were ten years of practising family medicine and my diploma in sport medicine, which I was certain would come in very handy during my deployment.

On the first day, I found out that my ID card, my Geneva Conventions card, and my security clearances were out of date. What a way to start things off! Despite this rocky beginning, I ended up learning a great deal during the following two weeks of training. This included learning how to throw grenades, fire rocket launchers, and shoot pistols, rifles and machine guns. During our weapons qualification training, I was initially given a standard-issue C7 rifle that did not have properly adjusted sights. On the shooting range, my first ten shots ended up nowhere near the target. While everyone else was "zeroed in" after their first ten rounds, it took me twenty-five. However, once my gun sights were properly adjusted, I managed to shoot one of the higher scores. To the dismay of my instructors, every time I was asked to do something very army, I would drop to the ground and give them several totally pathetic imitations of a one-arm push-up. This involved supporting myself with an absolutely straight right arm and jiggling my body around as though I was having a seizure. Before our training was completed, the staff were starting to expect this type of misbehaviour from me, and I did my best not to disappoint them.

We were also briefed on additional topics relevant to our deployment: the political situation in Bosnia, the rules of engagement governing our use of force while deployed, the international laws of armed conflict, how to do a rucksack march, foreign vehicle identification, welfare issues, financial benefits, immunizations and fitness training. Disconcertingly, our training also included instructions on how to survive as a hostage, how to avoid land mines and how to extricate ourselves from a minefield should we ever find ourselves in the middle of one. We were even taught how to start intravenous lines (IVs) and had to practise on one another. During the IV class, I quickly realized the safest option for me was to volunteer to help with instructing the practical part of this session. While none of my teammates managed to successfully establish an IV, at the very least I managed to avoid becoming a human pincushion. Towards the end of our training, our public affairs officer gave a presentation in which she informed us that the media was our friend and that we should not fear reporters or attempt to avoid them. Most of us were more than a wee bit skeptical, given that every day, it seemed, Canadian newspapers would feature headline stories about a new military scandal. Shortly following this briefing, military intelligence personnel gave a session in which they were very quick to point out that, above all else, we should never, ever trust the media. After that, whenever we saw our public affairs officer, we would repeat in a robot-like drone, "The media is my friend, the media is my friend!"

While I was in Petawawa, I was politely told that I shouldn't take a briefcase into a theatre of operations as it tends to make the troops nervous. A briefcase carried by an officer is a sure sign they are from National Defence Headquarters (NDHQ) and are there to provide help that is neither wanted nor needed. Acting on this sound advice, I bought a field satchel to carry paperwork, a combat field notepad cover, a combat business organizer (which I affectionately refer to as my "combat purse") and a wallet with the generic army "paint-by-numbers" pattern. I even had name tags put on them so I would appear to be even more "grunt-like." (Army personnel are commonly referred to as "grunts," particularly by Navy and Air Force personnel.) I have had several hard-core, knuckle-dragging trained killers salivating over my kit, but no matter how much they pleaded with me, I would not let them touch it – let alone use it. I am acutely aware that, although all this stuff is very warrior-like, more seasoned soldiers can identify me as a combat virgin from ten miles away. Perhaps if I got a few tattoos and shaved my head, I would stand out a little less.

While still in Petawawa, someone provided us with bookmarks that had Army propaganda on them – what a treasure! To show my gratitude, I put a small hole through the top of my bookmark and buttoned it onto the breast pocket of my combat jacket. I wore it all day, and when asked what it was, I proudly stated that it was my decoration of bravery for deciding to deploy with the Army. Those that didn't think I was insane before this training session are now absolutely certain that I am bat-shit crazy.

Not only was our pre-deployment training very educational, but it also allowed the National Command Element (NCE) personnel to bond into a cohesive team. This was important because I knew who I would be working closely with long before I left for Bosnia. When it came time to depart for Bosnia, I knew I wouldn't be standing alone in a line full of strangers dressed in the same uniform. Instead, I would be heading off to a strange new experience in a strange new country with a group of friends – this made a big difference to me.

When my pre-deployment training was completed, I realized I still had an enormous amount of preparatory work to do and very little time in which to do it: I had to take an Advanced Cardiac Life Support course (ACLS) and an Advanced Trauma Life Support course (ATLS), I had to have a full medical, I still had several equipment items to obtain, I needed to pack and send off my advance luggage, and I had to ensure that all of my patients were covered and my personal affairs were in order. Usually, it was expected that all of this would be accomplished while I was still working at my regular military occupation and my private practice. Fortunately, I worked for a good boss who understood the demands such taskings can make, and he told me to take the time I required to properly prepare for my deployment. His philosophy was that if the Canadian Armed Forces were going to task you, they should be prepared to pay the price to ensure that you have the time you need to get ready. Without his support, I would never have been able to complete all the things that needed to be done. As it was, my five weeks off before deploying were filled with so many obligations that it didn't feel like much of a holiday. I wish there had been more time to do some fun things with Janet and the kids. Perhaps it was a good thing that they were also very busy during this time.

By the late evening of the 11th of July 1998, my kit may have been ready to go, but my heart sure wasn't. It's hard to describe the deep ache you feel when leaving behind the precious people you have celebrated with for more than a quarter of a century of your life. You also realize that you will miss many of the one-time-only experiences that make a family stronger. I sincerely hope that my family understands what I am doing here and why I am going, because without them my life would have very little meaning.

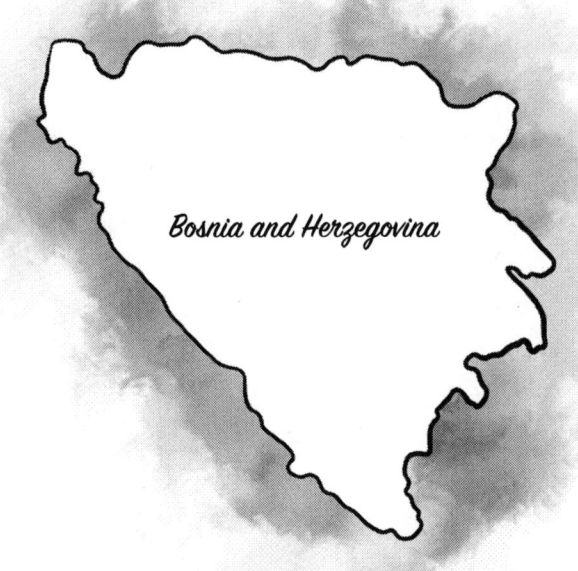

Bosnia and Herzegovina

July 1998

12 July 1998

D-day has arrived, and although I am somewhat excited, I also have grave reservations about what I have gotten myself into. While our plane is not flying out until 1900hrs, I had to report to Canadian Forces Base (CFB) Petawawa at 0830hrs the day before to ensure that I had everything I needed and that my luggage was properly loaded on a truck. I had to haul all my luggage to the farthest end of the building to be mustered, only to be told I had to haul it all the way back to the entrance of the building where it would be inspected, weighed and then loaded on the truck. I was then surprised with an agenda item that I did not expect – pepper spray training!

In April 1998, the city of Drvar saw the return of Serbs who had been displaced by the war. This sparked ethnic tensions which quickly elevated to murders and riots. It rapidly became evident that our personnel were not properly training to handle these types of confrontations, especially since all our weapons were designed to be deadly and could not safely be used to quell the violence. To provide us with a non-lethal defensive weapon, we would all be issued with pepper spray. The training to properly use this product involved a didactic lecture followed by a practical session in which we were able to taste the real spray, go into a room that had pepper spray in the air and then practise with simulators on each other. During the simulations, we were told to put one hand to the side and let our partners aim and shoot at the hand. I did as instructed, only to have my partner spray me directly in the face because she felt this would make for a more realistic practice session! Fortunately for me, the simulator is not nearly as disabling as the real pepper spray in a canister.

Once this training was over, I returned home to spend one last night with my precious family. This involved some long-distance driving, but it was totally worth it. Janet drove me back today, and in classic Darrell fashion, I arrived about two minutes before my name was yelled out during the roll call. Shortly thereafter we were marched out to the departure zone with a bagpiper providing the musical accompaniment. I got to hold my wife of twenty-three years for a minute or so and could not help crying as I knew how much I would miss her and the kids. Janet and I have said a lot of goodbyes during our life together, but this will certainly be the longest time I have ever been away.

Of all the days to fly out, they had to pick the day of the World Cup finals. Fortunately, we arrived in CFB Trenton just in time to watch the entire game and witness one of the greatest sporting upsets of the decade, when France won their first cup on home soil against the defending champions, Brazil. We finally took off at about 1900hrs, and I managed to sleep for most of the flight. I sure will miss my family and friends back in good ole Russell, Ontario. Perhaps they will miss me too.

———

13 July 1998

We arrived in Zagreb at 0900hrs and were met by a heat wave, that has been gripping this area of the world for several weeks. I was also met by the person I am replacing, Major Robin Harris MD, who has been here since 30th of December 1997. From our conversation, I understand he has had a very demanding deployment and is ready to head home to his family who have undoubtedly missed him a great deal. He and I will be very busy over the next few days, as we have many meetings to attend and a full handover to conduct.

The handover to me will be complicated by the fact that I have never been in a theatre of operations, and my experience working with the Army is rather limited. One of the first things that happened was that I was issued my Browning 9mm pistol and twenty rounds of ammunition. Even medical personnel are expected to be armed whenever they travel outside of the camp. As a physician, I find it very

difficult to have to carry a weapon, even though the Geneva Conventions allow physicians to carry weapons to defend themselves and their patients. I sincerely hope I never have to do this.

Every time we enter the base, we must "clear" our weapons in a special safe area called the "clearing bay." The aim of this clearing exercise is to ensure that people do not inadvertently have live rounds in the chamber of their weapons when they enter the camp. The Army takes this practice extremely seriously. If in the process of clearing your weapon, you accidentally fire off a round in the clearing bay – which is a safe zone – you will be in crap up to your eyeballs. The Army has a name for everything, and the accidental firing of a round is affectionately referred to as a "negligent discharge." To someone with a perverted mind, this could sound more like an act of self-stimulation than firing your weapon by mistake. It's a good thing my innocent mind doesn't work this way!

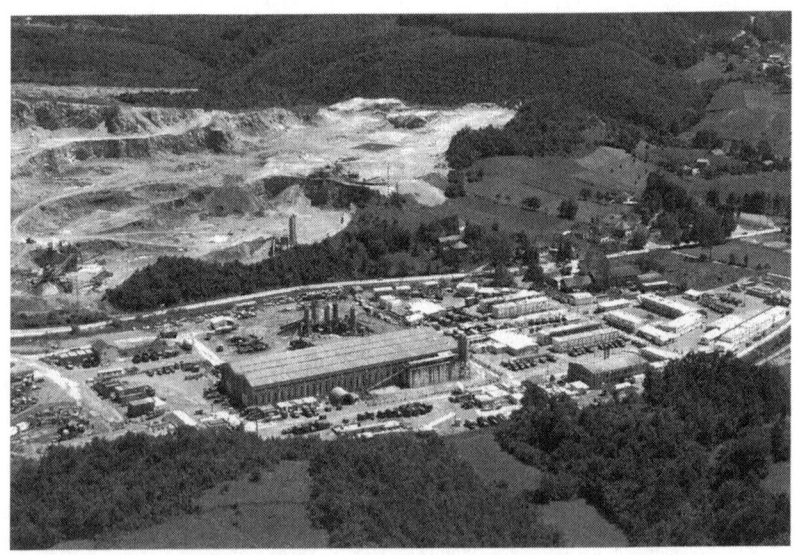

This aerial photograph of Camp Holopina (Coralici) demonstrates how "industrial" my new home for the next seven months truly was.

One of the big questions when you head off on a deployment is how much stuff to bring. The advantage of packing a lot of stuff is that it will help make the luxurious tin can that you live in a little more comfortable. The disadvantage is that you must haul this crap everywhere you go, and by the end of the day it starts to get very heavy. As a rookie, I elected to pack too much and ended up paying the price.

Before arriving at Camp Holopina, in Coralici, Major Harris said Coralici could be best described as "industrial," and he was absolutely correct! The camp is built around an active cement factory. There is an asphalt plant left of the front gate as well as several functioning quarries within throwing distance. On the positive side, just outside the camp are numerous rural trails that pass through some of the most beautiful countryside I have ever had the privilege of running in.

It has been a very long day, and I need to put my head down so that I can better meet the challenges that tomorrow will undoubtedly bring.

---

14 July 1998

Yesterday was a long day, but I managed to sleep very well despite the unique and very foreign environment in which I now find myself. My home for the next seven months will be a converted sea container that the Army affectionately refers to as an ISO (International Organization for Standardization). Given the name, you would think it would be called an IOS – just one of the many things about the Army that I will never understand. An ISO is essentially an eight-by-twenty-foot metal box with a door at one end and a small window at the other. As a senior officer, I am very privileged to have an ISO all to myself. Most of the personnel in the camp must share their ISO with at least one other person, which must certainly be very crowded and would most definitely afford very little privacy. My Army-issued interior designer ensured that my ISO was equipped with a bed, two desks, one chair, two stand-up metal cabinets and a lamp that does not work. Extravagance isn't a word that comes to mind.

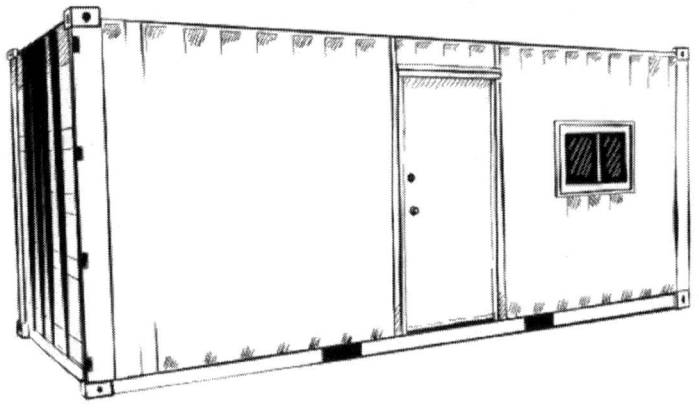

Home Sweet Home!

The camp washrooms have three shower stalls and while they do offer hot water, the supply is limited, and the temperature is set way too high. In fact, the water is so hot that a new arrival burned himself taking his first shower in theatre – welcome to Coralici! It appears that I will never share this young man's fate, as there isn't even lukewarm water available by the time I try to shower after my morning workout. It is hard to put into words the joy of taking an ice-cold shower after a hard run. If I am finding this unpleasant experience a challenge to my strength of character during the scorching heat of the summer, how bad will things be when I try to shower during the bitter winter months. I would be remiss if I didn't mention that to get to the washrooms, I must take a brief walk outside, which can present problems for me in the middle of the night when my aging prostate gland starts singing to me.

While I have very little to compare it with, the word on the street is that Coralici is the nicest of all the Canadian camps in Bosnia. If this is true, the rest of the soldiers in our contingent must be living in pretty spartan conditions. The meals are excellent, the exercise trails are super, the weight room is well equipped, the camp is not all crammed into a single building, and we have the Advanced Surgical Centre (ASC). Many of the soldiers find it reassuring to know that we have a Canadian surgical team in theatre, should bad things start happening again. Ethnic tensions remain high in Bosnia, so it wouldn't take much to have a return to the violence they saw during the war. The ASC is staffed with a commanding officer (CO), a general surgeon, an anaesthetist, operating room (OR) nurses, intensive care unit (ICU) nurses, an x-ray technician, a lab technician and a host of medical assistants. The OR looks as modern as anything you will find in Canada. The dilemma for personnel in a unit like this is that, while being busy would make the time go by faster, they hope for the sake of our troops that their services are rarely required.

I have broken down and bought an army-green eating utensils bag for carting cutlery, cups, bowls and plates to and from the mess hall. This is a very handy little item as it allows you to keep your hands free for practical things such as returning salutes, doing one-arm push-ups and scratching your bum.

---

15 July 1998

On our schedule for today was something referred to by the Army as a Board of Inquiry, in which the National Command Element (NCE) personnel were given a handover briefing in front of the entire staff. It was interesting to see how well the Roto 2 personnel had managed to morph into a well-oiled machine. I am certain these shared experiences help to form lifelong friendships for many people.

Major Harris and I continue with our own handover. There is so much to go over and so little time, that I can see the frustration on Robin's face. Robin is very handy with a computer, but I on the other hand, am far more comfortable with a pair of runners and a soccer ball. I am certain that more than half of the stuff he showed me how to do will be lost forever in the empty cavern I call my brain.

During my daily travels, I ran into the new Battle Group (BG) Commander, Lieutenant-Colonel (LCol) Jorgensen, who just happens to be a keen soccer player and enthusiast. He assured me that if the opportunity presents itself, members of our contingent will play friendly games with local soccer clubs and other contingents' soccer teams. If this works out, I hope to get a chance to be involved in one way or another.

I have started waking up at 0550hrs to go running in the cool of the day. It is impressive to see so many other military personnel doing the same thing. Based on the strange looks we are getting from the locals, I am certain they think we are lunatics – they may be right! In the evening, I have also started going for mental health walks with our Judge Advocate General (JAG) officer (legal advisor), our psychologist (PsychO), and anyone else who is desperate enough to desire our company. The exercise is great, the conversation is stimulating, and the view is magnificent.

---

16 July 1998

Today we attended the official transfer of responsibility for the Canadian Contingent Stabilization Force (CCSFOR) from Colonel (Col) Romses to Col Walter Natynczyk. A transfer such as this involves a formal signing-over process. As they were signing the documents, Col Romses ended up having to wait for Col Natynczyk to finish. When Col Natynczyk noticed this, he attempted to explain his slowness by saying, "Mine is longer than yours." It was only after the entire room erupted in laughter that he realized what he had said could easily have been taken in several different ways. Being a good sport, he took it all in stride, but for the remainder of the ceremony, his complexion remained a little redder than usual.

Today was the last day that my predecessor spent in Coralici. I thought he would have been more excited to be leaving, but he looked completely exhausted. What I did not fully appreciate was how much more he and all the other personnel who were heading home were going to have to endure before being reunited with their families. First, they must pack up all their kit and load it into containers that will accompany them. Then they have a long hot bus ride to headquarters (HQ) in Velika Kladusa (VK) where they get to spend a long time standing in line waiting to be processed. Then they get to set up their own cot on the gymnasium floor for sleeping. The next morning, they get to travel to Zagreb where they await the plane heading home. When they finally return to Canada, they get to spend three hours on a bus before they reach CFB Petawawa where they must go through a "clearing out" process before they can go home to the arms of their loved ones. This doesn't sound like something any overtired soldier would look forward to going through.

With Robin's departure, I was finally able to arrange my living space and working area the way I wanted it. It continues to amaze me that an office never quite feels like it's yours until you change a few things around – even if those changes have nothing to do with increasing the efficiency of the place. My wife refers to this process as peeing in all the corners to clearly mark your territory. I intend to take my time with this project and make at least one small improvement every day for the foreseeable future. Making this place seem homier will be a real challenge, and I hope I have enough urine to do the job properly.

17 July 1998

We have been in theatre for five days now, and today was the fifth time I had to be at the National Command Element HQ in Velika Kladusa for meetings. This is making it very difficult to get settled in either my office or my quarters. While the two camps are only thirty kilometres apart, it takes forty-five minutes to get from one to the other. When we travel by road, we cannot exceed sixty kilometres an hour, and the fines are very heavy for those caught speeding. Imposing a speed limit seems unnecessary as the roads are very narrow, serpentine in pattern and cluttered with farmers riding horse-drawn carts. SFOR (Stabilization Force) personnel are required to travel in pairs, and both soldiers must be equipped with their weapons, helmets, load-bearing vests and flak jackets. This bulky equipment can make going anywhere rather cumbersome, but in a crisis situation, it could save your life.

It is a happy day for the troops as the Contingent Commander has removed the alcohol restriction typically in place when the responsibility for the contingent is changing hands from one group to another. The alcohol consumption policy here is very straightforward: each soldier is limited to two beers a day, which must be opened in front of the bartender and consumed within the Mess. No one can accumulate beers that they do not consume or share their daily ration with another soldier. Drinking alcoholic beverages off the camp is prohibited for any reason. The joke is that your first two beers cost you DM2 (two Deutsche Marks) each, but your third will cost you $2,000. They are very serious about this policy, and it has virtually eliminated any of the alcohol-related incidents that have occurred in previous deployments. Some soldiers feel the policy is too harsh, but many other nations have similar if not harsher policies. It is important to remember that we are living and working in a potentially hostile environment and that being impaired by alcohol could cost you or your buddies their lives.

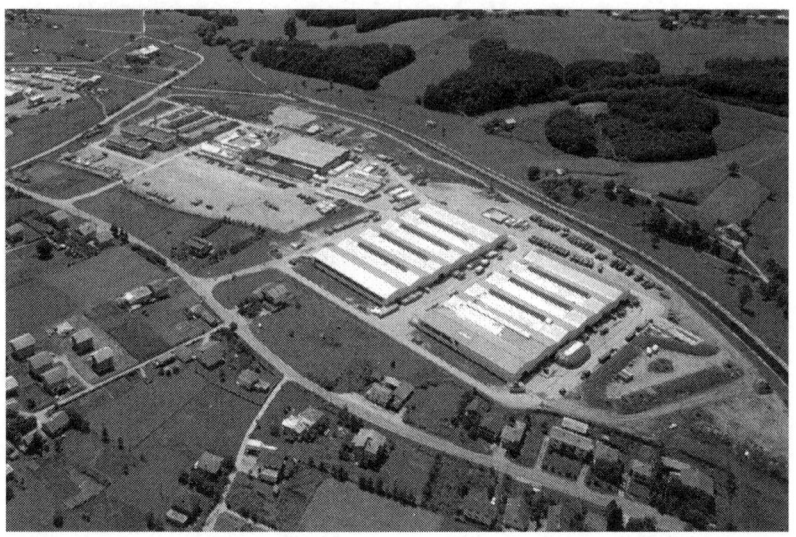

**Camp Veleka Kladusa (VK) was the largest Canadian camp in Bosnia
and home to our National Command Element.**

Today my predecessor will fly home to the family he has been separated from for nearly seven months. When we said goodbye yesterday,
he looked exhausted and in need of a much-deserved rest. I hope that
he gets to enjoy some hard-earned leave with his wife and children.

----

18 July 1998

Today I discovered that Saturdays in a theatre of operations are
like any other day of the week. This makes it difficult to stay oriented
to the passage of time – perhaps that is intentional. Camp Holopina
is built around a cement and brick manufacturing plant that was not

operating until recently. Much of the infrastructure in Bosnia was destroyed or damaged during the war, and efforts to rebuild could not begin until there was a formal ceasefire agreement. As the country begins to rebuild, materials are in demand, and the manufacturing plant is becoming more active. Greater use of the plant has two effects on our camp: it increases the volume of dust and fumes in the air, and it creates a great deal of noise. The machine that makes the bricks is very loud and begins operating at 0450hrs every morning. I am convinced that this is part of a scheme the locals are employing to make our lives more miserable while we are here. I have started sleeping with earplugs, which seems to be helping. I feel sorry for the Advanced Surgical Centre staff whose quarters are immediately adjacent to where the brick-making machine operates, as they must find it impossible to sleep even with earplugs.

The volume of dust and fumes in the air has also raised concerns regarding the quality of the air our soldiers are being exposed to. After considerable effort, we were finally able to get a British air quality assessment team to visit our camp. As luck would have it, it rained for most of their first visit. On the one day that it didn't rain, the wind was blowing the fumes away from camp, so a proper assessment could not be completed. Fortunately, the team will be coming back to repeat the assessment – this likely has as much to do with the fact that we treat them like royalty when they are here as it does with the fact that we really want the assessment done. Apparently, the standard of living in our camps is much better than that of our British counterparts.

Today was the first of the Battle Group Commander's weekly meet-ings. These are frustrating events, as I swear that the participants do not speak English. The language spoken could best be described as "Army" and it consists almost entirely of acronyms, slang and abbre-viations. The scary thing is that I am beginning to understand some of what is being said. Hooah!

During the meeting, we were informed that, as part of the peace-enforcing process, the warring factions have supposedly been disarmed, and these arms are warehoused in special monitored areas referred to as "cantonment sites." These sites are inspected frequently to ensure that what is supposed to be there, actually is there and remains there. Despite this effort, we heard two bursts of automatic weapons fire on our evening fitness walk. We reported the incident and were later informed that there was a wedding in the area, and the discharging of weapons is a traditional part of the festivities.

---

19 July 1998

Every Sunday we have "Sunday Routine," whereby all personnel who are not performing operationally essential tasks get to relax and do whatever they want to until 1300hrs, and then it's back into uniform. Even this early into the tour, such a tiny gesture of normalcy seems very important – for without it, one day drifts into the next. I celebrated the day by sleeping in and going for a run on the "club" route at 0700hrs. Someone on the Army staff had gone through the effort to map out a number of running routes so that soldiers would have some idea of where they were going and how far the run would be. This particular course has a hill on it that seems to go on forever and ever (seventeen minutes to be exact), but when you finally reach the top and are successfully resuscitated, you are treated to an incredible view of the mountains that surround the area. The view is almost as breathtaking as the climb, and you find yourself wondering how the people who have been blessed with this beautiful homeland could have so much hatred for each other that they would risk destroying it all.

Today was my first day on call, and we ended up admitting a young man whose tour of duty is just ending, and he has what appears to be an acute gastroenteritis. He tried not to report to the hospital, but his abdominal cramps were so bad that he simply could not function. He did not want to disappoint his family by returning home even later than scheduled, especially since he had already given up an earlier flight so that one of his men could head home a little earlier. The soldier is actually quite ill, and the surgeon is concerned that he may have a perforated bowel due to diverticular disease. He required an IV but was so uncomfortable and apprehensive that the staff could not find a vein to insert the IV catheter into. They called me in to help, and while I have only started one IV in the last eight years, I didn't let anyone else know this. I approached the patient with outward confidence and internal apprehension. With a whole lot of help from God, I was able to insert the catheter on the first try – something both the patient and I greatly appreciated. I hope he is OK. I can't imagine the disappointment his family will experience if his return home is delayed due to his illness.

---

20 July 1998

We were up at 0600hrs to take a four-and-a-half-hour journey to Sipovo to visit the British 5th Field Ambulance. The trip was a never-ending collection of winding narrow roads and switchbacks through some of the most beautiful countryside you will ever see. Unfortunately, the beautiful scenery is frequently marred by homes that have been burned down or blown up. The region between Bihac and Sipovo experienced some of the most extensive fighting during the war, and in their efforts to ethnically cleanse the area, the warring factions destroyed entire villages. The area is still heavily mined, and hardly anyone has attempted to move back. It is amazing what people can do to each other.

On the way to Sipovo, we stopped at Camp Maple Leaf in Zgon to pick up Captain (Capt) Jim Chung MD. He is the senior medical officer (MO) in the 3rd Royal Canadian Regiment (3 RCR) Battle Group. This is where the majority of the "ground pounders" (infantry soldiers) in the contingent reside. The soldiers in Zgon are crammed into a small factory and live under canvas that has been set up inside the factory. The camp is well laid out but is a little more tightly packed than I personally would like.

The field ambulance in Sipovo has some 235 British medical personnel who are also living under canvas inside an old carpet factory. They have two operating theatres and a complement of surgical staff. Personnel within our area of responsibility (AOR) who require orthopaedic or trauma surgery can be medevaced to them via Sea King helicopter. They are not very busy these days, and one of the major issues for their leadership is finding ways to reduce staff boredom. One way of doing this is to have staff exchanges with other contingents – we may be able to arrange something with them.

Our patient in the ASC with the acute abdomen is less uncomfortable but continues to have an elevated band count – a marker for infection. I hope that the triple antibiotic therapy he is on will reverse this trend and that he doesn't end up having to have abdominal surgery. Unfortunately, this young man was scheduled to head home tomorrow, but his long-awaited reunion with his wife and kids will have to be delayed. This must be very difficult for his family who have not seen dad for over six and a half months.

21 July 1998

Today was by far the hottest day of our tour with the temperatures reaching 42°C. The effect of the heat is amplified by having to work in full combat clothing in sea containers with little to no airflow.

I continue my efforts to improve the appearance and efficiency of my office. The JAG's paralegal bought me a nice flowering plant and the addition of a little greenery into my workspace has made all the difference in the world.

I ran the "heart" route this morning with Captain Fil Edora, MD, and we covered the eight-kilometre distance in 30:10, which is really moving given the hilly nature of the route. I would like to run it in twenty-eight-something before our tour ends.

The food here is quite good – it's easy to imagine soldiers going home having gained a fair bit of weight. Our soldiers are kept very busy doing patrols, standing guard and training. I am impressed with the professionalism of our service personnel, but some might not agree if they based their opinion entirely on what they read in the newspaper headlines back in Canada.

At the Battle Group Commander's "Evening Prayers" (Army slang for an evening meeting), I noticed a young major who looked vaguely familiar. Before the meeting ended, I realized that he was the son of an old friend and that I had coached his little brother's minor hockey team thirteen years ago. It is moments like this that remind me I am indeed getting a little bit older. I already miss being with my crazy family, and every once in a while, I resent that I will never get back the time I spend here, to spend with them. Knowing that this is true for everyone here doesn't make it any easier to accept.

Our patient seems to be finally coming around. For the first time in five days, he has been able to eat and keep his food down. He is looking forward to heading home. Praise the Lord.

---

22 July 1998

This morning our camp was rocked by an explosion – I wasn't sure if we were being shelled by enemy artillery or not. The entire place shook as if an earthquake were taking place. As it turns out, the rock quarry across the highway from our camp does some intermittent blasting, and only greenhorns like me worry that something bad is happening.

The temperature rose to 42.3°C today – I was dripping wet just working in my office. I can't imagine how miserable it must be to work all day long doing patrols in an armoured vehicle while wearing a flak jacket and load-bearing vest.

I spent the morning working in the unit medical station (UMS) as Captain Edora was out doing a recce (reconnaissance) on a local medical clinic in which he hopes to do some humanitarian work. I got to see three patients with very minor problems, none of which were sport medicine related.

In a rare act of courage, I made my way to the local barber. This was a frightening experience as every man who leaves her shop has virtually no hair left on the top of his head. To add to my concern, the guy exiting the shop as I was entering pulled me aside and suggested I go somewhere else because the barber wasn't in the mood to cut today. If his haircut was any indication of the barber's mood, I would have said she was into taking scalps. It took me several minutes to muster up the courage to trust my follicularly challenged head to a stranger armed with scissors and clippers, but I did, and she ended up doing a great job. While I would describe my haircut as somewhat shorter than usual, it is still a far cry from some of the Kojak trims favoured by the "sharp-enders" (a slang term meaning the military personnel who work at the front lines).

The latest military intelligence reports indicate that the situation in Kosovo seems to be deteriorating, and this has the potential to create instability in our AOR. If things really get bad, we may even be sending some of our troops and medical assets to Kosovo. I hope that calmer heads prevail soon. Warrant Officer (WO) Bergdahl is our senior medical assistant – her husband returned from Bosnia in January '98 only to see her deployed to the same area in June '98. From the sounds of things, he is likely to be deployed again before she even returns home. Perhaps these types of situations are why the CAF used to advertise that "There's no life like it." You can say that again.

---

23 July 1998

Today has been a long day, and as I write this, I am very tired. For starters, the temperature reached 43.1°C, and once again you begin to sweat just thinking about exercising.

Early this evening we admitted to the ASC a forty-three-year-old soldier who had collapsed on a run two days earlier and has been having difficulty breathing and some chest discomfort. His electro-cardiogram (ECG) shows changes suggestive of an inferior wall myo-cardial infarction (MI – a heart attack), and he has an elevation in his serum cardiac enzyme levels indicating possible damage to his heart muscle. We decided to have him "airevaced" (medevaced) to Zagreb for a cardiology consult and a treadmill exercise stress test. Teeing up an airevac takes a great deal of work as you have to talk to people from all over the theatre, and they all want some piece of information that you invariably do not have at the time. I hope for this gentleman's sake the tests confirm that nothing is wrong or that we caught his condition before he sustained any major myocardial muscle damage. He does not appear to be very happy with us as he feels that there is nothing sig-nificantly wrong with him. Unfortunately, this kind of denial is all too common, especially in a macho organization such as the Army.

My office is really coming along. I now have a map of the AOR with little markers indicating where our camps are and the time it takes to fly to each. This is the kind of stuff you see in war movies. Hooah! I have a picture of my family on my computer and seeing their tanned and smiling faces makes me wish I were home enjoying their wonderful company. I even miss Baby, our somewhat insane Siamese cat, and her antics.

Canadian troops were part of an operation that just captured several persons wanted for war crimes in the former Yugoslavia. Everyone was very pleased with this mission, but the persons who were captured ended up being released because the legal authorities did not have sufficient evidence to proceed any further. This was frustrating for everyone. I am amazed at the volume of intelligence work that our troops do to ensure that we have a good grip on what is going on in our AOR. Every day it seems that someone is trying to get away with something. This week the mufti (an Islamic legal expert) of Banja Luka passed away, and since then there have been clashes between various ethnic groups in that city. The contingent has banned all CAF personnel from travelling to this area for any reason until things settle down.

I hope that tomorrow is cooler and quieter.

---

24 July 1998

Yet another scorching day in the former Yugoslavia with the temperatures once again in the 40s. I had a great workout this morning and am actually beginning to enjoy running on the hills here.

Today was a bit overwhelming for me as I had requests for both my time and opinion from many different directions. One of the priority concerns appears to be the sale of bodybuilding supplements such as creatine and protein powders in the unit kit shops. The concern is coming from the very top and has to do with the potential liability to the Crown for condoning the use of products that could be potentially harmful to our soldiers. Amazingly, they have this concern for the sale of creatine but not for the sale of tobacco products. I looked at some resource material that I brought with me, surfed the Internet and talked to some subject matter experts to find out that creatine does seem to work, and research to date has failed to demonstrate any significant adverse effects.

I have started playing soccer with members of the Battle Group's soccer team. The only downside is that we have to play on a cement parking lot that is covered with a fine layer of dust and the odd rock or two. Call me old-fashioned, but as a goalkeeper I refuse to dive on concrete, and this hinders my ability to play the position well. I would be remiss if I didn't mention that a sizaeble lack of talent also hinders my ability to be a good goalkeeper.

We had our second meeting of the National Command Element today and it appears that Col Natynczyk is very concerned about the

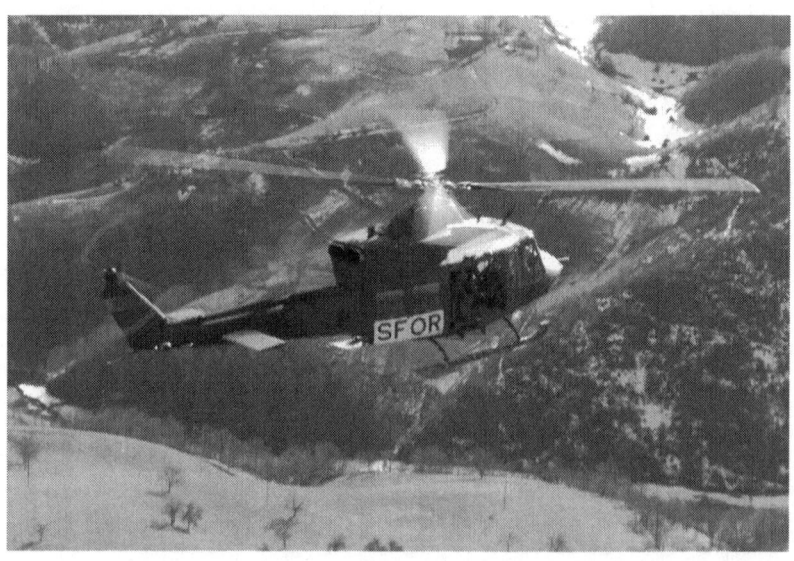

A Bell CH-146 Griffon Helicopter flying over the hilly territory in Canada's area of responsibility. They were an excellent addition for the mobility of our contingent.

welfare of his troops in Bosnia. The Canadian government has finally agreed to deploy three Canadian helicopters and their support staff to CCSFOR. These birds will certainly improve our ability to move around in the AOR and will finally give us our own air evacuation capability.

Our patient who was airevaced to Zagreb could not get all his tests done today and so will have to remain in the hospital over the weekend. He will not be thrilled about this, but his unit will be sending personnel to keep him company during what will probably be one of the longest weekends of his life. I only hope that all his tests can be completed by early this week.

The local economy has literally been destroyed by the war, and now the unemployment rate is approximately 70 percent. While this is staggeringly high, the people who live in our rural area do not appear to be starving. Most of the farmers we see still manage their land primarily with manual labour, which may explain why not many locals appear to be obese. I would really like to spend an evening watching a movie with my loved ones.

---

25 July 1998

Saturday is a working day in theatre, and this takes a little getting used to. I have decided that I will try to keep Saturdays as quiet as possible so that I have an opportunity to recharge my batteries for the demands of the coming week. I spent most of the morning researching and writing the Commander's briefing note on the use of creatine monohydrate. I enjoy looking at these kinds of issues, and I hope that the Boss finds it informative.

The temperatures remain in the 40s and today we had our first person present with heat exhaustion. He was given intravenous fluids and admitted to the hospital. Considering the hours people work here and the fact that we are all unaccustomed to these conditions, it is surprising that we have only seen one heat-related injury so far. We have been encouraging the leadership to ensure that their soldiers drink enough so that their urine remains clear. I know the message has been passed on because every so often a soldier passes me in the camp and says, "Don't worry sir, my urine is still clear." In turn, I inform them that the sharing of this very personal information will help me sleep better at night.

Tonight, the cooks prepared a surf and turf supper with lobsters flown in from PEI. There is no doubt in my mind that Canadian soldiers are the best-fed soldiers in the theatre. While my wife is a wonderful cook, I don't normally eat this well when I am at home, and I am sure this is true for many others.

As the Commanding Officer of the ASC, Major Langlais has a tremendous amount of responsibility. She has twenty-three people working for her and all the headaches associated with running a mini hospital. She is very well-organized, very conscientious and clearly focused on taking care of the medical needs of all CCSFOR personnel. She is a great team player, and I think we will work very well together.

Our contingent psychologist, Major Charlie Fournier, returned from a trip to Sarajevo today. He was not impressed by the amount of destruction that he saw and the areas that are still unsafe to visit because of land mines. What a pity, as I had always imagined Sarajevo as a beautiful place to visit. Sarajevo is home to a very large German field hospital in which they have a neurosurgeon and almost every other specialty you can think of. Once we get our own helicopters, sending people to this facility will be considerably easier.

---

26 July 1998

Today was the first time I had the opportunity to go to Mass while in theatre. As with everything in these kinds of camps, the chapel has been constructed by combining three sea containers and functions as a classroom the rest of the time. We have 330 personnel in camp and managed to have seven soldiers attend Mass. It takes a little getting used to, seeing the minister saying Mass in his combat uniform. We have an Anglican minister based out of Coralici where I am located and a Roman Catholic priest in Zgon. They will switch around every so often so that everyone will get a chance to attend a Mass in their own faith. It is remarkable to see how similar the Anglican and Roman Catholic Masses are. The minister introduced a nifty little music machine that can be programmed to play all kinds of hymns. After several attempts we finally got the tempo of the music adjusted such that we did not have to sing at one hundred miles an hour.

The first Contingent Commander's conference for his commanding officers was also held today. Out of necessity we had to cram over thirty people into a room designed to hold a maximum of twenty. The fact that the air conditioning was not working properly did very little to help the four hours pass any faster. These sessions are important, but when you have to attend most of the briefings, much of what is covered has already been repeated two or three times. When the meetings are over, everyone wants to talk shop with you, and I ended up heading home two hours later with enough work to keep me busy for the next week. The Commander wants us to get out and see the AOR so that we more fully understand what we are dealing with. I wholeheartedly agree with him and can see that arranging for travel while still dealing with all the other demands will help to make each day pass quickly.

I have been practising my left-footed kicking and ball-handling skills. I have already seen some improvement and I hope with six and a half months of practice I can get to be a much better soccer player.

Janet's first set of care packages arrived today, and she sent a small radio/CD player and this sure makes the office a nicer place to work. The Smarties and jujubes were a nice touch and should keep me from going through sugar withdrawal while I am here.

27 July 1998

Today, much to my surprise, I was asked to join some soccer players from Coralici to play indoor soccer against a team from VK. I was scheduled to be on call for work but managed to switch the schedule and plan my day around this much-anticipated opportunity to have some fun. Before departing, I had to inform the Commanding Officer of the Battle Group that the cardiologist in Zagreb had completed the assessment of one of his soldiers and concurred with our diagnosis of an inferior wall MI. This also means that the soldier must be repatriated back to Canada for further tests and treatment. The meeting was about to conclude just in time for me to grab my soccer stuff, hop in the back of a two-and-a-half-ton truck and head off with the team. As I got up to make my departure, the CO indicated he wanted me to be available at 2000hrs to answer any potential questions the patient might have. Duty calls once again, and my plans for soccer went up in smoke. While I understand that my role in theatre is to try and provide the best care for our soldiers, this was still disappointing.

On today's morning run we came across a pair of four- or five-week-old kittens that had been left on the roadside. They were curled up together on the canvas bag they had been abandoned in. They looked almost as helpless as I felt at that moment. The large number of animals roaming freely on the streets suggests to me that the people in this area have given up on animal control for the moment. I guess when you are trying to rebuild your country, pet control would be fairly low on a very long list of priorities.

While the ASC is an important contingent asset, it seems that most of the personnel have no idea what it can do. To address this lack of understanding, the ASC had an open house today, and personnel from all over the AOR came to see what services the centre has to offer. It was nice to see so many people come through and good to see the staff get an opportunity to strut their stuff. The ASC's Commanding Officer also used the event as an opportunity to impress upon the senior leadership the need for specific improvements such as teleradiology.

We saw a young soldier with pneumonia today, and it was interesting to assess him clinically, review his radiographs and blood work, and examine his sputum under the microscope. Using all of the above and a CD-ROM of Harrison's Principles of Internal Medicine, we were able to make the diagnosis of streptococcal pneumonia.

------

28 July 1998

It is Nathan's twenty-second birthday, and I am too far away to slip home for some cake and ice cream. It helps bring some things into perspective when you consider that the average age in the Battle Group is only twenty-one.

After five days in the Sisters of Mercy Hospital in Zagreb, our soldier is still only getting daily ECGs and is going through culture shock: his cardiologist speaks very little English; most of his meals are spartan and unidentifiable; his medications are delivered in plastic pop bottle caps; and his urine samples are placed in pill bottles – to name but a few of the differences between the level of care he has been receiving and the Canadian standard of care. His unit is providing him with incredible support. He has had friends with him throughout his stay, and their daily supply of store-bought food is likely the only thing that has kept him from succumbing to starvation. The Army really does a good job of taking care of their personnel in these types of situations.

Given that the soldier has remained stable throughout his hospital stay, and the cardiologist has confirmed our diagnosis and has no more tests planned, I decided to go get him and bring him back to the ASC where we could monitor him while he awaits his airevac to Canada on the 2nd of August. Making this decision turned out to be easier said than done. I had to travel to Zagreb in a Bison ambulance (an armoured vehicle) with a crew of five medical people. Our Bison ambulances are built for patient extraction from the battlefield, and they are noisy, cramped and hot. They also have so many things hanging from the roof that you have to wear your helmet or risk being rendered unconscious during your journey. The normally three-and-a-half-hour road trip to the hospital ended up taking five and a half hours because we got lost in downtown Zagreb (some things never change). It was very frustrating as we saw our rendezvous point about one and a half hours before we arrived there. We made one wrong turn, but Zagreb's road system is set up in such a way that we had to drive another thirty kilometres down the road before we could turn around. To add to our misery, we managed to get lost a second time. This kind of stuff seems to happen to me quite often. When we finally met our soldier, he was sitting on the hospital's front steps. He told us that as soon as the specialist found out we wanted to take him back today, his bed was given away, and he was left unattended for nearly seven hours. By the time we got back to Coralici, our trip had taken ten hours, and everyone was tired – especially our patient. It was a good learning experience for me, but

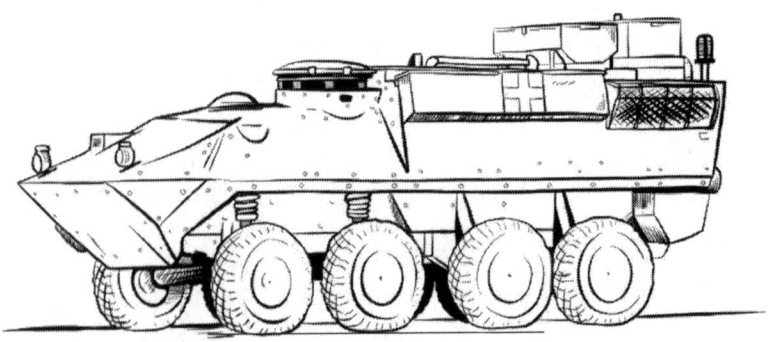

A Bison Armoured Ambulance

unfortunately, it came at the expense of one of our troops. Major Langlais has been handling the mountain of administration needed to ensure his air medevac back to Canada, and she looked exhausted when the day was finally over. In this environment, it is amazing how much work it can take to ensure that our patients are properly cared for.

---

29 July 1998

Today I had the opportunity to visit the Battle Group's Platoon House in the city of Bihac. I am told that during the war, Bihac was under siege for one thousand days. The town's inhabitants are almost entirely Muslim, and they refused to surrender to the Serbs. Although Bihac is no longer a hot spot, the Battle Group has a detachment of thirty-two soldiers who live in two poorly protected buildings in the middle of Bihac. Their role is to show a military presence and to monitor the many weapons cantonment sites that are in the area. The medical facility they have is very small, and four men are forced to live in the same area as the examining room. This makes it difficult to provide patients with even a small amount of privacy.

The soccer team was all excited today because we had an opportunity to practise on the local soccer pitch. We only had forty-five minutes on the field before the hometown team arrived and wanted to get onto their field. We politely left the field and then spent an hour watching them practise and getting totally psyched out. I must admit, sitting there in the sun without a uniform or weapon, I almost forgot I was in war-torn Bosnia. Sports truly are a great outlet. We will be playing this team in four days, and based on what I witnessed, we will be hard-pressed to challenge them. Many of our players have not kicked a soccer ball in more than four weeks. It felt great to play again, but I have a feeling that the team has already selected its goalkeepers, and I will likely get little if any game time. I am hoping that I will not come out of theatre without having learned some new soccer skills.

The medical and food services staff have developed a mutually beneficial relationship. Every week, the medical team helps unload the huge volume of food it takes to feed this camp, and in exchange, the food services staff provide us with some Gatorade and other goodies. Today I was able to help with the unloading, and now I don't feel quite so guilty when I help myself to a Gatorade. To combat the extremely hot weather, the Commander has obtained a huge volume of bottled water and Tilley-like combat hats for the troops. These measures have proven to be very effective, as the ambient temperatures have been considerably cooler since these items were delivered to the camp.

Our lawyer just returned from a liaison visit at a new rest and recuperation (R&R) centre that we will be trying out this rotation. He described the place as paradise, with virtually every sport you can imagine, a five-star hotel, lots of cultural centres, and an active nightlife. The only people who can afford to go there are the wealthy, and the mayor describes the town as a peaceful haven for anyone in need of a rest. I don't think this town has any idea what is about to hit it when our lads descend upon them for some much-needed unwinding after being stuck in theatre for six weeks. The mayor told our lawyer that the town has existed for over fifteen hundred years and survived many conquering invasions. I can just imagine the newspaper headlines after we arrive: "Town survives Genghis Khan, Caesar, Hitler, and Lenin but is completely decimated after one week of vacationing Canadian peacekeepers." I think the best move would be to go with the first group to visit because we will most likely never be invited back.

----

30 July 1998

Life here has been so busy that I cannot believe this week is almost over. This is probably a good thing, as it helps the time go by more quickly.

While this theatre is much safer than it used to be, it is still a dangerous place. The other day, a team of Belgian soldiers went off the road in their armoured personnel carrier – two were seriously injured and regrettably one died. The roads here are very narrow, and the civilian drivers are absolutely crazy. Today we were travelling down a narrow mountain pass with a rock wall on one side and a river on the other side, when a semi-trailer truck drove by and missed side-swiping us by about six inches. Shortly after, while returning along the same road, we found that the same semi-trailer truck had tried to pass an armoured personnel carrier, and both vehicles ended up damaged. Fortunately, no one was injured. Much of our travelling today was along either the Una or the Sana Rivers. Both rivers are gorgeous, and it was difficult to watch the local people enjoying a refreshing swim knowing that we could not partake in such a refreshing summertime pleasure.

Today there was a bombing in the region and several people were killed. Houses continue to be set on fire in the Drvar region and there are reports of possible forced-labour logging camps. The entire region seems to be controlled by powerful mafia-type leaders, and much of the violence we see is all part of a well-orchestrated intimidation campaign aimed at discouraging refugees from returning to areas from which they were ethnically cleansed. With the elections fast approaching, we anticipate there will be an increasing volume of these acts of intimidation. Much of the Battle Group's work is focused on intelligence-gathering so that we can defuse problems before they get out of hand.

Janet finished the last clinical day of her nurse practitioner program and sounded very relieved on the phone. She has worked extraordinarily hard to complete her program, and I am extremely proud of her. I wish we could have celebrated this special day together.

31 July 1998

Today started with a road trip to Banja Luka for a meeting of all the senior medical staff in the Multinational Division Southwest (MND/SW). No one in the vehicle had ever been to Banja Luka, and once again a two-hour-and-fifteen-minute trip managed to take us four hours. The available maps are of poor quality, and the roads are devoid of directional signs. To add to our problems, CCSFOR personnel are only allowed to travel on routes that our engineers have deemed to be safe – this means that the risk of encountering a land mine is lower but still isn't zero! On the trip, we passed towns where nearly every home had been destroyed during the war. Now the few remaining houses just stand there as a silent reminder of how powerful a force hatred can be. The meeting was great, as we had the opportunity to meet our British, Dutch and French colleagues. Unfortunately, the Czechs could not make it. We were able to discuss in detail the medical services available in the AOR and to share our mutual concerns. It was interesting to note that the British are also unhappy with the poor quality of care available in Croatian medical centres and only use them as a last resort.

I was on call last night and was busy for a change. We had a patient from VK admitted with lower leg cellulitis and the staff could not get his IV started. Once again, I was fortunate to be able to get things going. That's two for two – but then who's counting? We also had a sinusitis and a knee injury. Our last patient slipped and fell into the razor wire that surrounds our camp, and his left hand sustained multiple lacerations. I elected to sew him up in the OR, and it took eighteen stitches to close his deeper wounds. These types of injuries have a good chance of becoming infected. We'll need to watch him closely.

The Deputy Chief of the Defence Staff (DCDS) will be arriving tomorrow, so there is considerable excitement in the camp. It seems that over the next month we will be visited by a whole bunch of people who are high up on the food chain. This will keep our senior staff

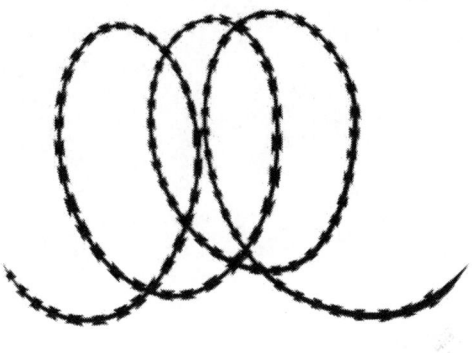

Razor wire

much busier than they want to be. Apparently, the Surgeon General is scheduled to come and visit for the first time ever this fall. It will be good for him to see firsthand some of the limitations that his medical personnel are required to work with on a daily basis.

August 1998

1 August 1998

The 40-plus-degree weather continues to plague the Coralici area, and I must admit that having to wear full combats in this kind of weather can be very unpleasant. It was especially uncomfortable today as Lieutenant-General (LGen) Crabbe came to visit our humble camp, and everyone was told to remain in uniform until he left, which was sometime after 1900hrs. The Battle Group had a parade for him, briefing sessions, dinner in the officer's mess and finally a night patrol.

Today was clean up my room day. I cannot believe how quickly it becomes a mess with only me throwing things around – and all these years I thought it was Janet.

We had a patient admitted to the ward with mononucleosis and the lab tech took me aside and showed me how to identify atypical lymphs and band cells. I must confess that I really enjoy looking at things under a microscope.

As we work here, the role that different organizations play is becoming increasingly clear to me. We still have a lot of details to iron out, but with a little cooperation, things will eventually run smoothly.

Our contingent lawyer has become known as "the Candy Man of Coralici." When we go out for our nightly walks, he brings a bag of candies with him, and the kids run out to meet him with their hands out and big smiles on their faces. It seems like such a small gesture, but it says so much about who he is and in many respects mimics on a smaller scale what Canadian soldiers are trying to accomplish here.

Our ASC staff have taken on a project to improve the local surgical facilities available in Bihac, a town about forty-five minutes south of our camp. Some of their equipment is damaged and our medical equipment tech will attempt to repair it. The surgical suites are equipped with air conditioners that haven't worked in a long while and are well beyond repair. As a consequence, during this heat wave the surgeons are inadvertently dripping sweat directly into their patients' wounds, which does little to reduce the rate of post-operative infections. Hopefully, we can find the money to get them the number of air conditioners they require. Bosnia could use a great deal of help rebuilding, and if we can keep the warring factions from destroying themselves, it just might happen.

I really would like to have a quiet evening at home with my loved ones, but for now, I will have to content myself with looking at their beautiful faces in the pictures I have stuck to my computer.

2 August 1998

It is now 2200hrs, and my office still feels like an oven. This may have a lot to do with the fact that today's temperature reached an unbeliev-able 43.7°C. This would not have been so bad, but the 3 RCR soccer team had a game to play against a team from one of the local towns. When our team arrived at the stadium, we found out that our opponents would be high school-age boys. These youngsters played hard for the full ninety minutes, and despite the sauna-like weather, they didn't even appear to sweat. This was the first opportunity I had to meet the 3 RCR goalkeep-ers, and both are very talented – much more talented than I will ever be. The game ended in a 1–1 tie, and this was only possible because both keepers made a number of absolutely outstanding saves. It was interest-ing to note that while they both have very different styles, they were both very effective. Any dreams I may have had of playing net for these guys dissolved as I watched their current keepers perform. I did get to warm up with them, which is more than I expected to be able to do on this tour, and for this opportunity, I am truly grateful.

The Roman Catholic chaplain celebrated Mass with us today. I find it such a privilege to be able to attend Mass while we are here. I hope we will be able to do something special to celebrate Christmas. Perhaps we could build a manger with scraps of wood available in our camp.

While we are lucky to have it, the phone system in theatre could drive a saint to swear. First of all, there are a limited number of lines available, so when you dial someone the number almost always rings busy. When you are lucky enough to finally get through, you often get a bad connection and a time delay that makes having a normal conversation almost impossible. I have spent the entire day trying to contact someone at our camp in Drvar and simply could not do it. I am now beginning to realize why they call Drvar the "black hole."

My running partner decided not to train today, so I had to do my workout inside the confines of the camp because we are not allowed to go outside the wire alone. This isn't much fun, but it sure beats sitting around on your rear end all morning long. People saw me go by so often they were getting dizzy, and I am certain by now they are convinced that I am a nutbar – and they are probably right.

---

3 August 1998

The heat continues, and today it seems to have sapped me of a great deal of my usual energy. There was no soccer scheduled for tonight because all the players were feeling quite beat up from yesterday's game. The Canadian Forces (CF) have established a welfare fund to buy the soldiers some nice-to-have things – to make life in theatre a little more tolerable. Courtesy of this fund, our camp recently took charge of fourteen new mountain bikes. These should be hot items for the short time that I predict they will remain in one piece. Can you imagine a bunch of testosterone-laden grunts riding a bike that belongs to someone else, up and down the mountain trails that we have around here? I give the bikes two weeks maximum before they are unserviceable.

We continue to have to wear our full combat uniforms in this weather while other countries allow their personnel to work in T-shirts. It seems that everyone is afraid that if our soldiers are allowed to work in T-shirts, it will trigger some kind of common-sense revolution, at which point the Army would be in real trouble. It's moments like this when I realize that the old Canadian Forces recruiting motto proudly stating, "There's no life like it!" never actually tells you what kind of life it is, only that there is no life like it. I can't say they lied. Hooah!

---

4 August 1998

This morning as we were standing at the gate to the camp, I overheard one of the guards telling someone that they had run the heart route in a good time of 35:00 but that one of the soldiers held the course record at 28:00. I can't explain why, but I felt challenged by this. Early into my run, I realized that I was feeling very good and decided to go for the record. It was very hot and humid, but I managed to run the course in 26:47. This has created a bit of a stir around camp. How will the Army ever deal with the fact that some ancient Air Force medical major can run faster than any of them? I must admit that I was very pleased with this performance, as one of my tour goals was to run the heart route in less than 28:00. I will now set my sights on running this route in under 26:00.

I finally had the opportunity to teach one of the in-service training sessions to the medical staff and I really enjoyed it. My presentation was entitled "The Practical Examination of the Knee," and I tried to make it as down-to-earth and relevant to the audience as possible. From the comments I received afterwards, it appears that I accomplished my mission.

The intelligence personnel continue to document minor problems throughout the AOR: citizens possessing weapons they should not have, SFOR road signs being torn down and anti-SFOR graffiti being written in public areas. While the theatre is much calmer than it once was, the CCSFOR leadership is reminding everyone to remain vigilant because little problems could easily develop into major problems in a short period of time.

We have a Canadian serviceman in Sarajevo who is not coping well after seeing some anatomical specimens at the university that he apparently found to be very disturbing. I spent the much of the evening talking to people before advising the Commander that, in my opinion, this soldier needs to head home as soon as possible. It always amazes me how complex repatriating personnel seems to be. It is easier to deal with these problems when I remind myself that what we are trying to do is protect our soldiers from further harm. I pray that our medical team can live up to this goal.

----

5 August 1998

Today we had our first real break in the weather, with the humidex making it feel like only 20°C. My body was a little beat up from yesterday's maximal running effort, so I took it easy and really enjoyed my workout. I have got to do more arm work if I hope to accomplish at least a single one-arm push-up before the tour is done.

Today was the first time that all the general duty medical officers got together in one place and discussed a number of professional issues. The meeting was very useful for me, and it addressed several concerns we all shared. I am very fortunate to be working with three wonderful individuals. Although they do not have a great deal of military experience, they are learning very quickly.

I finally managed to play an indoor soccer game with our team. Our opponents expected to beat us handily and were quite upset to find themselves bowing in defeat. It was a lot of fun, and I hope to get more chances to play in the future.

The Canadian contingent recently received our shipment of paint-by-number military hats that will keep the sun off our faces much better than our berets. While all the other units have begun wearing them, the troops in Coralici have not, and I suspect this is because the leadership in the Battle Group doesn't feel that these very practical hats look good with a combat uniform. As a result, our paint-by-number hats are being held in storage for as long as possible. Being a troublemaker, I procured one of these hats from another unit and will begin wearing it around the camp tomorrow. I am sure such a bold move will be greeted with some overt displeasure. I am starting to feel very comfortable in my combats, and I will regret not being able to continue to wear this very practical order of dress to work when my tour of duty is finally over and I return to the National Defence Medical Centre.

---

6 August 1998

Today was the most comfortable temperature wise since we have been here. You could actually wear your uniform and not perspire just sitting still. The PsychO, the JAG and I decided that today we would wear our camouflaged sun hats, which we affectionately refer to as our "combat sombreros." Man, were we unpopular. The soldiers were so taken aback by this break from military tradition, that they were virtually speechless and treated us as if we had leprosy. We could not have received more negative attention if we had walked around camp buck-naked.

A major walked into the mess this evening, his face and neck badly sunburned. When I offered to lend him my combat sombrero, he was very adamant that despite looking very much like a boiled lobster, he would never, ever, over his dead body be caught with that hat on his "Army head." Unfortunately, this is the kind of "resistance to change" style of leadership that has our young soldiers doing all kinds of stupid, dangerous and illogical things simply in the name of military tradition.

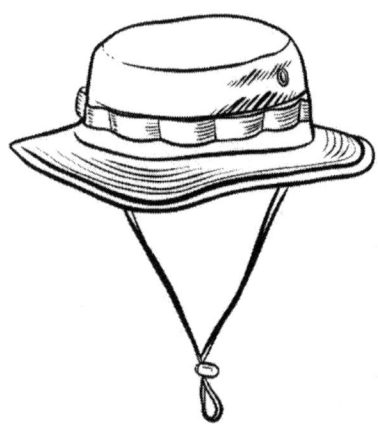

The much-maligned combat sombrero

One thing that working in this theatre has taught me is that no one has a monopoly on stupidity. At today's intelligence briefing we were informed that some communities are experiencing desperate shortages of water. In one town, the citizens were reduced to drinking mud, while their mayor owns a fleet of trucks designed to haul water. To date, their mayor has refused to haul any water because he's upset that he has to register his vehicles. To help deal with the crisis of stupidity, Canadian troops ended up having to deliver water to the town. The mayor is very likely part of the mafia that has a firm grip on almost everything that happens in this area of the world.

As well, we were told that the warring factions have finally admitted that the riots in Drvar, where several Canadian soldiers sustained injuries, were all staged to send a "Don't come back!" message to the people commonly referred to as DPREs (displaced persons, refugees, evacuees). The message must have been received loud and clear because only a very small percentage of the expected DPREs have returned to their homes this year. As the elections approach, we are likely to see more frequent actions designed to intimidate anyone who is thinking of returning home to live or vote.

I've only been in theatre a month, and I am already beginning to see some folks at National Defence Headquarters (NDHQ) as out-of-touch paper-pushers who have no idea that the entire reason for their existence is to support the soldier in the field so that he or she can perform better. I sincerely hope that I don't forget the lessons I am learning here because never want to become one of those people. I miss laughing with my family. I hope that God is taking good care of them while I am away.

----

7 August 1998

Life here has begun to heat up again as predicted. At 0130hrs, someone in Velika Kladusa shot a rocket-propelled grenade (RPG) at the Democratic People's Union (DNZ) headquarters. The DNZ is one of the national political parties, and it appears that someone is trying hard to discourage people from voting for them. In anticipation of retaliation by the DNZ, the Battle Group moved a lot of firepower into our Velika Kladusa camp. Everyone here has a real sense that this is only the beginning of the troubles, and we still have five more weeks until the elections are held. To add to all the confusion, NATO (North Atlantic Treaty Organization) has announced that if Serbia launches another offensive against the Albanians, then NATO will retaliate by launching offensive strikes against them. This is a risky strategy, as the Serbs are backed by the Soviets, Ukrainians and Greeks. Once again there is talk of shifting Canadian ground forces around in the event of a full-scale war. I hope for everyone's sake this does not happen.

Yesterday, the PsychO, JAG and I had a "hero picture" taken of us in our combat sombreros standing beside an Iltis vehicle (basically Volkswagen's version of a Jeep). This morning at the Contingent Commander's intelligence briefing, it was announced that one of the citizens wanted for war crimes in the former Yugoslavia was being facilitated in his efforts to escape justice, by three nefarious characters. We were also informed that our intelligence personnel had been able to photograph the trio for easy identification by our troops. When the picture was flashed up on the screen for all the staff to see, it was entitled "The Three Amigos" and featured the PsychO, the JAG and me doing our hero poses beside the Iltis vehicle. A good laugh was had by all. I am certain that we will forever be labelled the Three Amigos.

The Chief of Police reported that one of our armoured vehicles had accidentally hit and killed a cow on the road several days earlier. He reported that the owner was now trying to "milk" the system with claims that were "udderly" ridiculous. He emphasized there was a lot at "steak" here and that the entire issue was a bunch of "bull." This also got everyone laughing.

Despite the joviality, everyone is looking quite tired these days. All the build-up to getting here, then a month of working till 2300hrs every day can get to you. This arduous deployment work schedule is pretty much the same as my usual work schedule back home, so working these hours doesn't bother me as much as it does some of the other personnel. People are going to have to learn how to pace themselves or they will burn out quickly.

One of my running buddies will be out for the next two months with a stress fracture that we diagnosed this afternoon. We will miss his

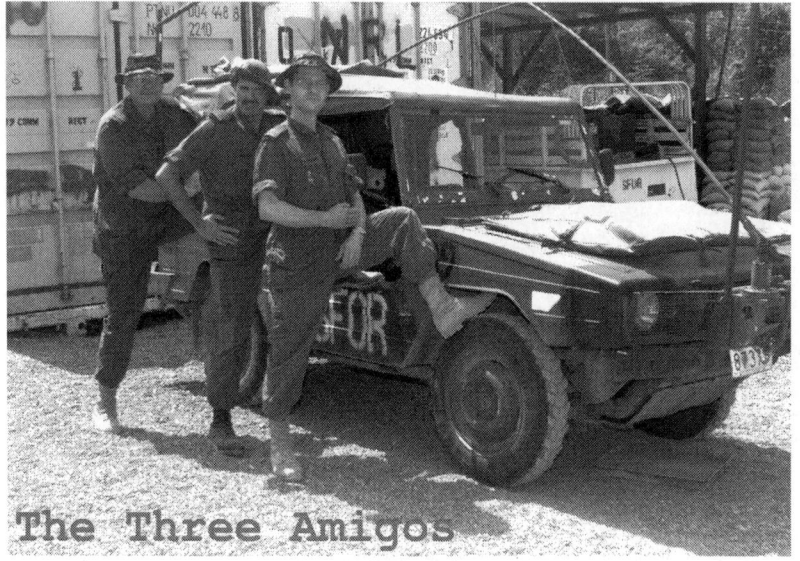

The Three Amigos

**From left to right: Major Charles Fournier (Psycho), me (Doc) and
Major Sylvain Lavoie (JAG) posing in front of an Iltis vehicle in the
new "combat sombreros" that the hard-core Army personnel hated.
The troops labelled us "The Three Amigos" and we loved it.**

smiling face at our morning workouts. Seeing him in the clinic reminded me that we will soon start seeing an increase in overuse injuries in
some of our personnel who are training much harder than usual.

———————

8 August 1998

We left at 0600hrs today to visit the Dutch and German hospitals to
see what services and what quality of care they can offer our patients.
There were five of us travelling with all our weapons and personal

protective equipment, so believe me when I say our vehicle was crowded and hot. Our map recce showed that if we took the "amber" route, we could potentially save a great deal of travelling time. What a mistake that decision turned out to be. The amber route ended up being a logging road that winds its way up one side of a mountain and down the other. It is single lane, covered in loose gravel, with many potholes – some the size of craters. We didn't see another vehicle for seventy-five minutes, and there were no houses anywhere in sight. What we did see was mine tape and several completely demolished buildings. This was the first time since I have been here that I truly felt uneasy. For whatever reason, I was concerned we might be ambushed and that it might be days before anyone found our remains. When we finally arrived at the Dutch hospital in Novi Travnik, their surgeon informed us that he, too, had made the same journey at night and would never do it again. The Dutch hosted us well, and their surgical centre is outstanding. It is spacious and very well laid out. The Dutch have the same two beer a day maximum rule but take a much softer approach to fraternization.

From Novi Travnik we went to the German hospital in Rajlovac, which is a suburb on the outskirts of Sarajevo. This facility is staffed by over four hundred personnel and is essentially a big city hospital that just happens to be located in a dilapidated old building. The facility has a CT scanner, a neurosurgeon, an ENT (ear, nose and throat specialist), a psychiatrist, a neurologist, five ultrasound machines, a mass spectrometer, a laboratory bigger than our entire hospital, etcetera, etcetera. Surprisingly, most of their staff speak excellent English, so communication was relatively easy.

After having supper with the Germans, we travelled on to Camp Butmir – a multinational camp built on the edge of the Sarajevo airport. There is a large American military presence in this unit, and the camp looks more like a fairground than a military installation.

They have an enormous PX (Post Exchange – a military retail store) that sells very little aimed at stimulating the brains of its customers – things such as books, word games, puzzles. I can't help wondering if the American leadership fear that if their customers start using their brains too much, there will be a mass exodus from the US Army. They had an eighty-three-piece orchestra play a concert the night before we arrived and have scheduled a rock concert for the day we leave. They even have outdoor cafes and pizza places. I have heard several people say that US troops never go anywhere without taking America with them. In my opinion, you miss a lot of what the rest of the world has to offer if you take that insular approach to life.

In the evening, I once again got to do my workout walking along a barbed wire perimeter fence and slept in my uniform on the couch because I had made the mistake of assuming our hosts would provide us with beds – what a rookie.

---

9 August 1998

We were up early and hoping to see downtown Sarajevo and the infamous "Sniper Alley" before we headed home to "Stalag" Coralici. Sniper Alley was the informal name given to the main boulevard in Sarajevo, which was lined with sniper posts. Many innocent people lost their lives on this deadly stretch of road. Unfortunately, no SFOR personnel were permitted to go into town today, but we were not told why. Despite the restriction on our wartime tourism, we did get a depressing glimpse of some of the damage done during the intense fighting that occurred in this famous city. It is unbelievable to see the near-total destruction of the residential area surrounding the Sarajevo airport. There are apartment buildings with their facades completely blown off and the telltale pockmarks left by thousands of machine gun rounds decorating the outer walls that remain. What was even more amazing to all of us was the fact that people were still living in some of these apartments – life does indeed go on, but it must be a depressing place to return home to after a hard day at work. The return trip to Coralici took us nearly eight hours. Virtually every building we saw along the way was riddled with bullet holes.

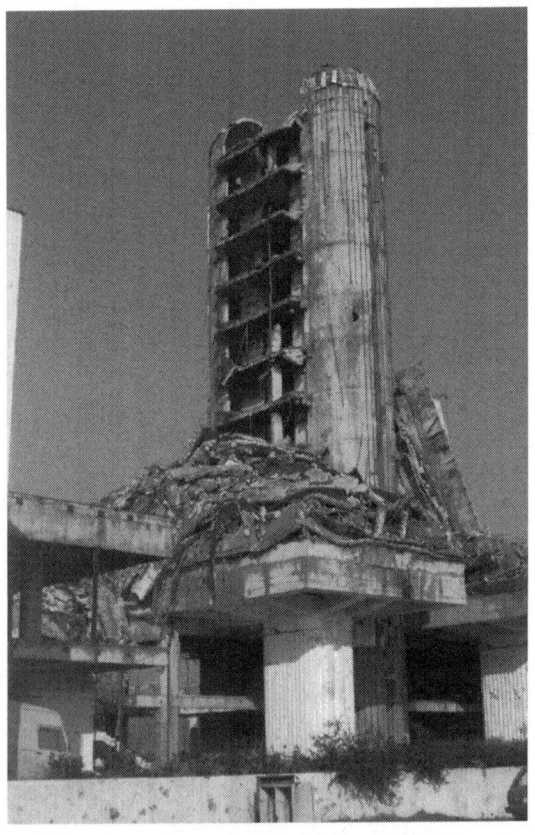

The Oslobodenje newspaper building after being pummelled by tank and artillery shells. Despite the massive damage, the staff continued to publish newspapers throughout the war.

A ten-kilometre road race was held in Banja Luka today, which I was unable to participate in because of our travels. The event took place at 1700hrs, and it was another scorching hot day. While no Canadian came away with any awards, some of our soldiers did run very well. The course was described as "brutal" because of the heat and the fact that the first five kilometres were entirely uphill. Maybe I will eventually get an opportunity to race later in the tour.

While I didn't physically exert myself this weekend, I am quite tired, which I suspect can be explained by a combination of factors including the heat, the lack of downtime and all the travelling I have been doing. The R&R periods are starting this week, and everyone is looking forward to getting out of uniform and having some time off to cut loose. When our soldiers are on R&R, they can drink and party as much as they want. I can hardly wait to see the repercussions of getting to enjoy these brief periods of freedom. The PsychO describes our in-theatre lifestyle as being consistent with that of a minimum-security prison, and the longer I am here the more I am inclined to agree with him.

---

10 August 1998

The first crew of folks just left for their much-anticipated R&R break. Only the Army can find a way to make what is supposed to be a break from the stress of living in a theatre of operations, a stressful experience. The troops who are departing must do so in full uniform and formed up in three ranks for the roll call. The troops then get bused up to VK where they get to sleep on the gym floor before heading out early the next morning. You quickly learn that if you elect to go somewhere far away, you will spend two of your four R&R days travelling on an un-air-conditioned bus. The departure trip isn't too bad because no one is allowed to drink until they arrive at the R&R

centre. The return trip is a potential nightmare depending on how hungover everyone is.

The AOR continues to remain hot in every sense of the word. Yesterday, someone threw a fragmentation grenade into a home in VK. In addition, there have been two incidents in which SFOR personnel were fired on – fortunately, no one was hit. To make matters worse, reliable sources of information are warning that threats are being made against SFOR personnel. The Commander of the Battle Group was not thrilled to hear this, and efforts are underway to minimize the number of targets we give terrorists the opportunity to shoot at. We have learned to expect acts of intimidation directed at Bosnian civilians, but everyone is somewhat surprised to see SFOR troops being targeted. For our personnel's sake, I hope this trend does not continue.

I am starting to settle into the rhythm of this place, making it possible for me to relax a bit more. This adjustment seems to conform to the graphs we were shown about how such taskings are experienced, where the first four to six weeks are characterized by excitement, the middle twenty weeks by boredom and the last four weeks by the excitement of seeing the finish line. I guess the trick is to try and find interesting things to do during the boring middle twenty-week period.

In the interest of reducing the incidence of motor vehicle accidents, SFOR has posted some ridiculously slow speed restrictions on the cleared routes in the AOR. Drivers caught violating these limits are heavily fined, as is the senior military person travelling in the vehicle. These speed limitations are so slow compared to the speeds at which the locals travel, that they are making our vehicles safety hazards. I found out today that the local citizens are starting to say that SFOR stands for "slow fuckers on the road" – the truth can be painful!

11 August 1998

The Battle Group for our contingent is made up of infantry soldiers from the 3rd Royal Canadian Regiment. I am starting to realize that if you are not a member of the Regiment, then you are somewhat of a second-class citizen in these camps. It is only natural for people to want to take care of their own, but it can be quite frustrating for those of us who are not members of the club. Simple things like office supplies, maps and basic furniture do not seem to be available when you ask for them, but you can't help but notice that they are still being delivered to regimental personnel. For the recent ten-kilometre race in Banja Luka, it was announced that the Battle Group would pay the registration fees and arrange transportation for their personnel only, and if there happened to be some room left over, it would be made available to non-regimental personnel such as medical staff. Now that I know the rules of the game, this doesn't bother me as much, but it can make tasks that should be relatively easy to do, much more difficult.

The mornings are finally starting to cool off, which makes for fabulous running. I am starting to meet some other good runners, and we should be able to keep each other company for the next few months.

Today is my thirtieth day in theatre, so I am now eligible to receive my tour decoration. Yeah! It is actually a nice ribbon, and my unimpressive looking uniform could use some more colour on it.

Today we met the recce group for the 408 Tactical Helicopter Squadron that will be joining the contingent this October. They will bring with them three Griffon helicopters and fifty personnel. The helicopters will certainly allow Canadians to move around the AOR better, and it will give us better airevac capabilities. They looked a little overwhelmed, and I rudely took the opportunity to share with them my thoughts on how they could best position their assets in theatre, without first asking them what plans they may have had. To their credit, they politely informed me that literally everyone they met thought they knew exactly what their squadron should be doing. After pulling my much cleaner foot out of my mouth, we were able to carry on with their visit.

---

12 August 1998

I am told that our joint task force (JTF) personnel will no longer take their vehicles into Croatia using Bosnian licence plates. Apparently, whenever they do this their cars end up being deliberately scratched, beat up or shot up.

We have an interesting laundry service here. Everyone is issued laundry bags and tags. You simply put your dirty clothing in the laundry bag and then secure it with a tag. There are pickup and drop-off times twice a day. Your laundry (colours and whites) is all done together, and I am told that by the end of your tour, everything ends up looking dull grey. I have also heard that people have had bags of laundry simply go missing, and while I felt sorry for them, I had some trouble personally relating to their loss. All of that changed tonight when I went to claim the two bags of laundry I had dropped off two days earlier and was told that only one had returned. The missing bag had two sets of combat pants, a personalized combat jacket and my cherished combat sombrero. I hope these items are eventually found because I am sure that replacing them will be an enormous hassle.

This evening, I watched a motion picture entitled *Welcome to Sarajevo*. The movie is a depiction of a true story, with real clips of the atrocities that were committed largely by the Serbs in the siege of this great city. I found the completely senseless and random killing of citizens to be very disturbing, especially since I had passed through Sarajevo less than a week ago and saw some of the damage firsthand.

We are currently dealing with several delicate issues including the technological challenges with implementing teleradiology and the proposed incorporation of our surgical assets into the UK medical facility in Sipovo. Everyone seems to have a vested interest in these projects, and it seems that we often forget that we are here to help the sharp-enders do their job better. Unfortunately, when the day is over and you close your eyes, you are often left wondering exactly who is supporting whom?

---

13 August 1998

After a few days of milder temperatures, Mother Nature has decided once again to bless us with extremely hot weather. We have only had one day of rain in the last five weeks, and I am not sure how badly this will affect the farmers' crops.

The local medical services here are dismal at best. I am told that if you have money, you will be well taken care of, but if you are poor or unwilling to pay, you will be ignored. Some physicians will not see patients from certain ethnic groups regardless of how ill they are – I wonder if they've ever heard of a little thing called the Hippocratic oath. Perhaps they took the "Hypocritic" oath. A lot of their hospitals' medical equipment is falling apart, but even if they had the money, they would still lack the support infrastructure needed to repair it. To illustrate just how bad things are, the hospital in VK has approached one of our medical officers about obtaining some tongue depressors because they have none. I can see being out of CT scanner film, but being out of tongue depressors is a little hard to swallow – no pun intended. If we get the opportunity, it would be worthwhile for us to sit down with the health care providers in the region to determine what their medical needs are, help prioritize them and begin working on fulfilling them.

This evening, the medical folks decided to have a basketball game. None of us are especially skilled, but we did have a hoot. The medics have named Captain Edora and me "Snake" and "Slime." I believe this is because he is so shifty on the court, and I sweat too much.

It is hard to believe that yet another exciting week here in Stalag Coralici is coming to a close. While people have compared being here to doing time in a minimum-security prison, I have noted two big differences. In the Canadian prison system, if you behave, the time you serve is reduced. In theatre, the worse you behave, the earlier you get to head home. In the Canadian prison system you can also enjoy a "conjugal visit"- good luck asking for that here.

Speaking of heading home, the first R&R period has just ended, and one of our soldiers is already in big trouble for getting drunk and throwing a glass out of a window where it landed on a car. The bodywork on the car will cost $1,500, and it won't surprise me if the soldier gets an all-expenses-paid holiday at the military's "Crowbar Hotel" in Edmonton, a place military personnel jokingly refer to as "Club Ed." These are the kinds of incidents that serve to reinforce, in my mind, the justification for limiting the amount that soldiers can drink while in theatre.

---

15 August 1998

I decided that today I would enjoy a little mini holiday here in Stalag Coralici. This involved not wearing my uniform at all, not shaving until noon, sleeping in until 0815hrs and spending two hours cleaning up the sea container I call home. While this may not seem like a whole lot, I felt great and really needed the break. The tragic part of this story is that I was only able to do this because of my rank and position. If I were a private deployed with this unit, I would literally go seven months without having to do much thinking because someone else would be telling me what to do every minute of every day.

LCol Paul Connelly arrived today to replace our anaesthetist who is being repatriated for medical reasons. It was funny to sit in the air-conditioned mess and watch LCol Connelly sweating profusely while those of us who had finally acclimatized were dry as bones. It will take him a few weeks before he can handle the 40-plus degree weather we are currently experiencing. The ASC staff said goodbye to our departing anaesthetist by shoving a piece of cake in his face and then dumping him in the toddler's pool they have set up in the back. To his credit, he took this in stride, claiming that the dunking solved two of his problems: the need to shower and the need to wash his clothes.

"Anaesthetist" is a very big word for some Army personnel to pronounce let alone understand. So, to make things easier for all our "green" clients, we have started referring to LCol Connelly as "Sleepy Doc." Yesterday the surgical team was operating in one of the local hospitals, and they had to take some infantry drivers with them to watch the vehicle and monitor the radio in case they needed to return to the ASC urgently. As luck would have it, a message did come through, and despite being briefed on the proper radio call signs, the only thing these two soldiers could remember was that one of the specialists was the Sleepy Doc. So, while our medical team was operating away on someone, they heard over the radio, "Sleepy Doc, this is mike one. Come in. Over"! I can only imagine what might have happened, had the Regimental Sergeant Major (RSM) overheard that transmission.

Most of the camp spent the day in Zgon for the Battle Group Commander's briefing. When they finally returned, everyone looked exhausted. I am happy I elected to have my mini holiday, even if it was spent behind razor wire.

16 August 1998

Nearly everyone was away this weekend, and the camp looked very much like a ghost town. This was actually nice because the tempo of life seemed to slow, and my body was telling me that I needed the break. Sunday Mass continues to be an intimate event, with only seven soldiers in attendance, and four of those are from the medical team. It is sad when you think that there is a captive audience of 320 people who live within one hundred metres of the chapel, and only 2 percent of them are willing to spend thirty minutes listening to the Word of God. I am pretty certain that I could draw a bigger crowd if I were to offer a lecture on how to safely use injectable anabolic steroids.

A huge thunderstorm rolled through this area and seemed to soak everything but Stalag Coralici. The camp could really have used the rain, if only to wash off the layer of dust that has accumulated from the operation of the cement and asphalt plants.

This morning, we ran the club route and once again had to climb up its monstrously long hill. I know I must be tired because the hill nearly did me in. Near the top, a dump truck slowly passed us, and I was very tempted to jump on the tailgate and hitch a ride to the top. The only thing that held me back was the fear that the badly beat-up truck would fall apart if I did this. You know you are in a world of hurt when you wish you knew how to say "Please shoot me and put me out of my misery" in Bosnian.

I continue to notice that there are two worlds in Stalag Coralici: the world that the Battle Group lives in and the world that we outsiders live in. The justice system is a good example. According to the JAG, it appears that the 3 RCR would prefer to deal with discipline issues on its own terms. Young soldiers have asked the JAG in private why certain infractions are always dealt with by assigning a heavy fine, regardless of whether they were accidental or due to negligent behaviour. The

JAG informed the young soldiers that this is not the way it should be. In response, they told him, "That may be all well and good, Sir, but what we are telling you is the reality we live in." I think it would be very educational to spend a month here as a private – it wouldn't be very much fun, but it would surely be an eye-opener.

---

17 August 1998

It was a sad day for the Army in Stalag Coralici. It seems that direction has come down from on high indicating that "Though shalt wear thy combat sombrero and like it," and the soldiers saw that it was good and complied. I knew something was up when I saw the Major who had said he wouldn't be caught dead in the paint-by-numbers hat, sporting his new chapeau around camp. When I met him, I couldn't resist asking when he had died. I don't think he thought this was as funny as I did.

Yesterday we had a visit from Brigadier-General (BGen) Holmes, the Commander of Land Forces Central Area, better known to me as the patron saint of running. He was in Trenton to see our plane depart for Bosnia, and we agreed at that time to go for a long run whenever he arrived in theatre. After looking at his schedule, I seriously doubt this will happen. I did get an opportunity to say hello to him during the twenty minutes that he was allowed to have for lunch. They then shuffled him off to a waiting helicopter to continue his tour.

Apparently, on the weekend, a reporter took a photograph of one of our airborne soldiers after being warned by him not to do so. The soldier responded by going into a rage and threatening to hunt her down and get even. While the reporter's actions were inappropriate, the soldier's response was way out of line. It will be very interesting to hear what happens to him – you gotta love those airborne fellas!

This evening, as a group of us left the camp for a fitness walk, we went by a dog that was sprawled out on the road and I commented, "I sure feel like doing what he's doing." Our anaesthetist responded to my comment by bursting into laughter. When I inquired as to what he thought was so funny, he informed me that when I made my comment, he happened to be looking at another dog on the road that was enthusiastically licking its genitals. I assured him that even if I was so inclined, I unfortunately lacked the required flexibility.

Over lunch today we found out that many of the young majors in the Battle Group are "acting majors," or in military speak, WSE (while so employed). This means that while they have not been officially promoted to the rank of major, they carry the authority of a major while they are employed in their acting position. The troops just call them "Velcro majors." This helps to explain a great deal about the dynamics in this organization, and I am sure this information will prove useful in the future.

I had the opportunity to meet some of the JTF soldiers today and they appear to have a fascinating career. These folks are the Canadian equivalent of the Navy SEALs. I would love to be involved with a special group like this, but they are frequently called away without notice, which has to be hard on your family life – not that being stuck here is great for one's family life either.

---

18 August 1998

Captain Edora and I started the day off by doing the "spade" route in a sizzling 36:19. I only kicked the last five minutes, and I am certain that I can run this course much faster if pushed to do so. It truly was a glorious morning to be out and sweating. My weight training is coming along in my effort to perform the elusive one-arm push-up. If Demi Moore can do it, so can I – I hope! She does have the advantage of having a much better-developed pectoral region than I do.

The unit medical station (UMS) has been participating in an exchange of medical assistants with our neighbours from the British contingent. Our unit has been blessed with the services of a young private whose nickname is "Chief." Chief spends the entire day walking around or sitting with such a vacant stare on his face, that you find yourself wondering if there is anybody home. Sharing my concern, the Sergeant decided to see just how vacant he was and sent him off to the supply section to pick up a box of fallopian tubes. To his credit, it didn't take Chief long to figure out he was being had. Rumour has it that Chief is sweet on one of our young female medics and I have a strong suspicion that he is in search of some fallopian tubes of his own.

The medical staff at NDHQ has decided to conduct a SIV during the election period. SIV stands for staff inspection visit, but I suspect it will more likely be a staff interference visit. CCSFOR has considered banning all visits during the election period to allow the Battle Group to focus on the mission. We will see what happens on this issue, but I can already see the sparks flying.

The meetings we must attend are getting shorter and more to the point as the novelty of being here appears to be wearing off. I am proud to admit that I now understand about 50 percent of what is being said, which is rather frightening. If this keeps up, I am worried that I may actually start to like it here.

I miss my family, our cats, our friends, soccer, the yard, cutting the grass and a whole bunch of everyday run-of-the-mill things. Dear Lord, look after my family while I am away. Amen.

19 August 1998

It has been a busy day in the war zone. This evening, we had a casualty evacuation exercise scheduled by the ops (operations) people. No one but the hospital warrant officer (WO), the CO and me knew this exercise was coming and that the brown stuff would hit the fan at about 1900hrs. The hospital WO and I headed out to the simulated accident scene and had a grand old time applying the makeup to our two victims. The ASC CO was departing the camp at 1900hrs for her three weeks' leave and was therefore unavailable. What no one else knew was that Captain Edora had scheduled his own casualty evacuation exercise for 1830hrs. When his ambulance crew radioed the ops centre to let them know that they were leaving the base to pick up casualties, the ops officers told them that they were cleared to leave the camp but should not have been told about the exercise beforehand. This caused a great deal of confusion for Captain Edora's staff because they had no idea what the ops centre was talking about. To make matters worse, when the ops people finally did contact everyone, they neglected to mention that this was an exercise. Everyone assumed it was a real emergency. Well, the quick reaction team came screaming down the road followed by an ambulance and an escort vehicle. A military police (MP) vehicle joined them with two very unhappy police officers who also thought they were coming to a real accident scene. The ASC also had no indication this was an exercise, and they fired up everything: rapid infusion pumps, IV lines, bear huggers, etc. Thank God they did not open the chest tube trays and other kits, or we could have wasted over $1,000 worth of materials.

The actual on-site medical assessment, management, evacuation and resuscitation in the ASC went very well. We truly do have very well-trained medical staff in the CAF. When everything was done, we went over to the ops people to ask why they had not informed everyone that this was just an exercise, and we were met by an arrogant young captain who refused to accept that he and his staff had screwed up. This will be a subject of conversation with the CO at tomorrow's briefing.

I had an opportunity to talk to the chief of surgery at the American field hospital in Tuzla. They also have a CT scanner and a very large surgical team. Apparently, the Americans are very paranoid about one of their soldiers getting injured in theatre, and so their personnel are confined to their camps and are not allowed to do any foot patrols. This sounds even more like a prison than Stalag Coralici. I have to close off for the night because the ambulance from VK is bringing in a soldier with a possible arm fracture.

---

20 August 1998

It has been a frustrating few days. I have been unable to get a telephone line to call home, even though I have two phones and access to a special line that is supposed to make it easier to call anywhere. Once again, I cannot imagine how difficult it must be for some lower-ranked soldiers to call back home to keep in touch with their families. Some of the bean-counters feel that allowing our soldiers to call home is a huge waste of money. I would like to suggest those REMFs (rear echelon mother$#!+&*%) try spending seven months here while also dealing with all the big and little problems that occur at home. It wouldn't take long before they would be singing a different tune.

We awoke to a beautifully warm rain this morning. Captain Edora and I were the only two people in the entire camp who went out for a run. It was very nice. As we came around one corner, we could both hear a funny sound coming from a sewer conduit. On closer inspection, I discovered a litter of kittens living inside the conduit, and they were very upset that their feet were getting wet. They were being extremely vocal, and it sounded to me like they were saying, "Help me! Help me!"

I had the opportunity to play two games of indoor soccer this evening in a neighbouring military camp. We won our first game and tied the second. The guys on the team are certifiably crazy and spent the entire trip stabbing each other in the back. It truly was hilarious to witness.

The injured soldier that came in last night was a Czech helicopter maintenance engineer, and he had a comminuted (broken in several places) and displaced Colles fracture of his left wrist. Funny as it may seem, we had absolutely no trouble getting a helicopter to take him to Rajlovac where he is due to have surgery in three days. I am afraid no matter how good a job they do, his wrist will never be the same. I also sent a Canadian soldier to Sipovo to see the UK orthopaedic surgeon. He will require open reduction and internal fixation for a displaced, rotated and intra-articular fracture of the base of his 5th metacarpal. Unfortunately, both of these soldiers will require RTM – return to momma!

I got to talk to Nathan tonight, and he strikes me as being much more mature than many of the young soldiers here in theatre. I hope he doesn't join the Canadian Armed Forces (CAF), as I don't think it would be good for him. He is going to apply to work with the Ontario Provincial Police (OPP) auxiliary force, which should give him access to specialized police training and may help him be selected to a police force in the future.

It is late, I am tired, and I need to wash up and call it another day. I miss my Janny B.

---

21 August 1998

The Rolling Stones played a concert in Zagreb last night, and apparently, some of our soldiers got to attend. You can bet that no one outside of a very select few ever got a chance to buy those tickets. These would have been well controlled by the regimental mafia.

The Commander jokingly noted that I appeared to be sleeping through some of his weekly briefings. Unfortunately, this is a very common occurrence for me, and I tried to reassure him that he shouldn't feel bad, as I had fallen asleep during briefings from individuals who were much higher up on the food chain and much more engaging speakers.

We had more excitement this evening. I had gone in to discuss a toenail excision with a patient when we got a call that a Czech HIP helicopter was bringing us a British soldier with an amputated arm, and the estimated time of arrival (ETA) was in thirty minutes. This was not an exercise – fortunately, the time we've spent in theatre has taught me to make phone calls to verify information. I called the MND/SW HQ to ask if they were aware of this airevac to us, and they said no, but they had dispatched their helicopter from Sipovo to pick up the injured soldier and take him back to their own orthopaedic surgeon. I then called our base in VK where the Czech helicopters are based. The staff confirmed that a Czech helicopter had indeed taken off and was intending to bring the patient to us. I then called the Czech contingent headquarters and was told that the Czech helicopter was already there, and the British helicopter would be there in five minutes. I asked them not to load the patient onto the Czech helicopter, as the British team would be there soon to take him home. In the meantime, we scrambled our ambulance and quick reaction force to the airfield just in case and put the ASC staff on alert. We were smart this time and did not open any perishable equipment. The drama lasted almost fifty minutes before we were finally stood down. I hope the soldier does all right. Somehow in this whole process, the patient with the non-life-threatening toenail problem was forgotten.

To burn off some of the adrenalin that we built up during the above adventure, we played one and a half hours of basketball. The basketball dudes (or "duds" to anyone who has seen us play) are slowly labelling everyone with a nickname. Our new anaesthetist, LCol Connelly, has been nicknamed "Sir Skid" because he wears worn-out shoes and is constantly slipping and sliding when he makes his cuts to the basket.

---

22 August 1998

As part of our regular operational training, we had a two-hour mine awareness lecture today. I learned a great deal more this time than I did when I had the lecture in April. I am sure this may have something to do with the fact that I am now living where an enormous number of land mines happen to be sitting in the ground just waiting to blow you up. It is truly scary to see all that human ingenuity being used to create weapons for the express purpose of killing and maiming people. Many of these weapons have mechanisms built into them specifically aimed at blowing up anyone who tries to disarm them. At the end of the session, we were taken out to a field with twelve mines and three pieces of unexploded ordnance (UXO) in it. My partner and I were able to find all fifteen items, but it wasn't easy even though we knew they were there. The combat engineers who were instructing us both had friends who had died in Bosnia because of these terrible weapons.

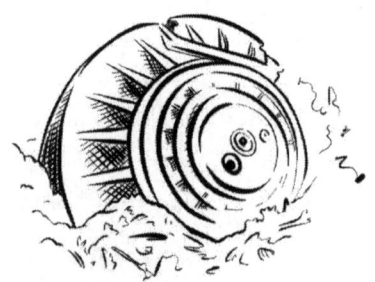

One of millions of land mines hidden in the Bosnian soil

I am noticing that fewer and fewer people are out for their regular morning run or walk – soon it will dwindle down to only those people who were training regularly before we left Canada. Some things never change.

Last night was the first time on this Roto that Canadian troops were shot at. The sniper was no marksman and missed by twenty metres, but that would have been close enough to get my undivided attention. At another location, a Canadian patrol was denied access to an area at a police checkpoint. The police had been drinking and apparently pointed their weapons at our soldiers. Showing the police the respect they deserved, our boys closed the hatch on their armoured vehicle and simply rolled right past the checkpoint.

To compound matters, today the SDA (Party of Democratic Action) and DNZ political parties are both having huge rallies in VK. There will be a lot of security personnel in place to try and prevent any sparks from igniting. I should also mention that the plum crop is now ripe, and the locals have their stills out and are making moonshine. This moonshine is like rocket fuel, and mixing a very potent alcohol beverage with simmering election tensions is like putting nitric acid and glycerin together. In anticipation of trouble, our state of alert has been increased and we must now travel wearing our flak vests. These things fit like a body cast and certainly do nothing to improve the comfort of our personnel during their daily drives.

In a briefing aimed at revealing the bigger picture, we learned that the Croatians apparently have their eyes on annexing a rather large chunk of eastern Bosnia. They are accomplishing this through a process referred to as "soft ethnic cleansing." Croatians have purchased all the major businesses in many areas and are only hiring Croatians to work for them. In many areas, residents are being confronted with threats of violence in a well-orchestrated effort to intimidate them into leaving or not voting. From what has been reported at the intelligence briefings, it seems that many people from many different places are just dying to grab a piece of Bosnia and make it their own. I have a feeling that SFOR will need to be here for a very, very long time.

---

23 August 1998

It is the end of week six, and I am still no less sane than when I arrived. I am not so sure the Army personnel can say the same because the Three Amigos have been working hard to make their lives miserable. Questioning the way the Army does business has almost become our unofficial mandate, and we love it. I am not so sure the Army would express the same sentiment.

Today our chapel was blessed by the donation of an altar cloth and religious banners from a parish in Newfoundland. It is amazing to see what a bit of colour can do to make a classroom look more like a proper church.

I had the opportunity to visit our camp in the town of Drvar. Drvar is located about two hours south of Stalag Coralici, in a deep valley surrounded by mountains. The town was badly damaged during the war, and many of the homes and businesses remain unoccupied. It is depressing to pass by big industrial centres and see all their windows shot out and their walls with huge holes blown into them. Our signals personnel call Drvar the black hole because it is very difficult to maintain communications with our personnel stationed there. This is very frustrating, as the communication lines have been down for as long as four days during our rotation.

Our camp in Drvar has 150 riflemen housed in the remains of an old grain storage facility and bakery. The troops have named the four main buildings after Canadian hotels. The main living quarters are referred to as "Castle Grey Skull." If you ever have an opportunity to see the main living quarters, you will be impressed with how appropriate this name is. The basement even comes complete with rats so large that the cats want nothing to do with them.

The UMS is housed within a modular tent structure within a warehouse and is the nicest looking UMS in the AOR. The senior medical person in camp is a 6B medical assistant (physician's assistant) and he is doing a very good job. At all these camps, the ingenuity of our soldiers is impressive. In Drvar, they have converted an old water bladder into a hot tub and painted palm trees on the walls to give it a tropical atmosphere. They have even built portable backboards that fit between two buildings and create the boundaries for a floor hockey arena. It is funny, but while I found nothing appealing about the camp in Drvar, the soldiers here appear to love it. Vive la différence!

We have started using live traps to catch the dogs that have been sneaking through the razor wire surrounding our camp. Most of them are skin and bones, and the locals do not appear to care about them at all. From the wailing that is currently going on outside, I would guess that we have caught another little furry friend who will be going for a ride tomorrow morning.

---

24 August 1998

The weather is definitely changing. The days are getting shorter, and the nights and mornings are becoming cooler. This is happening much faster than I expected it to. In the extremely artificial environment in which we are living, it is easy to forget that the school year is about to begin back home. I will miss the chance to see Matt and Jenny starting university – such a big milestone in life.

Today it seemed that every time I tried to accomplish a task, something would happen to make my original plan impossible. The one thing I did complete was the construction of a small wall shelf to hold my CD player and CDs. I have just finished installing it, and it not only looks great, but it also makes the office appear a bit more professional. The construction engineers allow me to use their shop and all the scrap wood I want. The shelf is primitive looking, and I have started to refer to the style as "early Coralici." The chance to work in the shop is a real privilege and I hope to build many more things before I have to return home.

The general practitioners had their second get-together this afternoon, and it is interesting to learn about all the humanitarian work that is being done by our contingent. The local area has a real shortage of physicians, as over half of them left during the war and are unlikely to ever return. The local cardiologist has an ECG machine that actually works, and he makes use of it whenever he can get his hands on the graph paper that the machine needs. Almost every civilian adult is hypertensive, and it is not uncommon to see blood pressure readings of 210/120. This is high enough to blow the top of your head off, and these people are going about their normal life untreated for this dangerous condition. I hope to meet with some of the local health care providers to see if CCSFOR can come up with a more coordinated approach to providing humanitarian aid in the AOR.

Life in the camp seems much quieter with 25 percent of our people away on some form of holiday.

We have yet another soldier on the ward with an unusual facial infection that is not responding well to oral antibiotics. I hope this doesn't continue for our entire rotation.

I just found out from a private that within a month of returning home, the Regiment is scheduled to leave for a major exercise that will take them away from their families for another four to six weeks – and the senior leaders wonder why many of our soldiers and their families are unhappy.

25 August 1998

Boy were we ever hit by a big storm last night. The wind threw the chairs outside my room around and it rained very heavily. It was so noisy that I had to put in my earplugs to be able to fall asleep.

This morning, we had the Battle Group Commander's briefing, and what used to be a ninety-minute marathon event took only eight minutes. The brevity was due in part to the Commander being away and to the fact that the AOR has been unusually quiet for the last three days. I hope this trend continues but I doubt it will last.

We were informed that our ceramic plates and real cutlery have just arrived. Up until this point, everyone who has ever served in this camp has eaten with his or her own field kit or with paper plates and plastic utensils. I should have known that as soon as I purchased my handy-dandy combat eating utensils bag, it would become obsolete. I think I will continue to eat with my field kit, just to bug the Army a bit more than I already do.

This evening, one of my basketball opponents was wearing a hockey jersey. As I was pressing up against him, I asked him why he was wearing something so warm to play basketball, and he explained that it functioned as his anti-slime shirt – to protect him from my excessive perspiration.

One of the soldiers in camp is a professional artist who is currently working on a painting that will be a collection of images from Roto 3. He is trying to include an action shot of as many of the various units as possible. From what I have seen, it will be an excellent souvenir of this tour.

Matthew had a tryout with the Carleton University varsity soccer team yesterday and I am dying to hear how it went. He is an excellent athlete, and I believe he is talented enough to contribute to most soccer clubs.

DIARY OF A DEPLOYED DOC

The surprise of the day turned out to be that my wall unit was still in one piece this morning. What also surprised me was that other seemingly normal people actually like it and have put in orders for me to make them one for their office space.

----

26 August 1998

The weather here has truly changed, and this morning I was tempted to wear a turtleneck shirt to keep warm on my morning run. You can really feel fall in the air.

During this morning's training session, the cutest little puppy came bounding out to greet me by the roadside. He could only have been a few weeks old, and it was so tempting to bring him home with me. This, of course, would have been impossible, as such impulsive acts are strictly verboten here in Stalag Coralici.

Captain Edora left this evening for his four days of R&R in the fabulous town of Porec. I hope he has a great time. I have convinced my professional colleagues to spend this evening in the pursuit of intellectual growth, and in an effort to achieve this goal, we signed out the Austin Powers movie. This is about as intellectual as I feel these days – which still puts me a few rungs up from the average WWF wrestler. Hooah!

I accomplished a great deal today and hope to do the same tomorrow. I will be covering the unit medical station for the next several weeks, which should slow me down somewhat. I am noticing that the chronic tendonitis in my left foot is returning now that I am running more and not cycling at all. This condition is a very good indicator that my running career will have some real limitations on it from here on in. It saddens me when I realize that my days of being able to run as far as I want and as often as I like are quickly coming to an end.

The Commander of CCSFOR has three designated advisors: the legal advisor, the psychologist and me. It frustrates all three of us when the junior staff ask us for advice and then ignore it or simply act without getting any advice at all. It is surprising to see how often they end up having to come back to us to try and straighten out the mess they've gotten themselves into by not listening to us in the first place. It is a lot like being the parent of a very large family – can you imagine being the mother of thirteen hundred grunts? It is a good thing that the Three Amigos have each other to vent our frustrations to or we would likely be mumbling to ourselves by now.

I would like to meet our new kitten whom the family has named Skye Blue. She looks as cute as a button, and I am told that our other cats Blue Boy and Bell are giving her a very rough time. Hang in there Skye, you'll soon be an accepted member of the Menard menagerie. Why any creature in their right mind would want to live in our bizarre household I do not know, but I welcome her just the same.

---

27 August 1998

Here's a news flash: the Army is beginning to suspect that soldiers may be having sex in camp – say it isn't so! The leadership suspects that the bunkers we use as shelters during attacks on our camp are also being used as shagging suites. The Three Amigos refer to this problem as "sex in the "COR.RI.MECS" (an Italian-made brand of modular buildings). Rumour has it that the Battle Group is considering having patrols check on the bunkers to discourage hormonally driven soldiers from using them to enjoy any carnal pleasures. If such patrols are initiated, they will likely be unofficially christened the "anti-shagging squads." I personally feel that whenever you have men and women employed together, in an isolated area, sex will become an issue. As long as individuals are discrete about their liaisons, I believe the Army would be far better off looking the other way and focusing their attention on the real mission.

The ladies' soccer team in Russell sent me a Zellers promotional T-shirt with a picture of Zeddy kicking a soccer ball on the front. I have been wearing it proudly around the camp, thinking that everyone would be envious of my splendid attire. This illusion was shattered today when one of the guys on the soccer team said, "Sir, while you obviously like that T-shirt, please do the team a big favour and don't wear it when we go to Rome." I can only assume he thought my precious teddy bear T-shirt lacked a certain army machismo.

With Captain Edora away for a while, I had the opportunity to see a good number of patients today. The one that stands out the most in my mind was a young military policewoman whose history strongly suggested a vaginal yeast infection. When the medical assistant who was doing her initial interview mentioned that the doctor might have to perform a gynecological examination, the young lady simply slapped the handle of her loaded pistol and said, "I don't anticipate that there will be any problems." This was so unexpected that everyone laughed.

I had another opportunity to play two indoor soccer games this evening, and we were fortunate to win both. I am finally starting to catch on to the unique way this game is played in VK's gymnasium. Once again, the entire team spent most of the trip trying to see who could insult the most people in the least amount of time.

Mother Nature seems to have a little surprise in store for Stalag Coralici – the winds are howling, and things are beginning to fly around again.

Dear Lord, please watch over all my family. Keep them safe in your loving arms so that I may once again have the opportunity to enjoy their hugs and kisses upon my return.

28 August 1998

The weather has gone from boiling hot to freezing cold in twenty-four hours. I actually had to put a sweater and sweatpants on to be comfortable. For the first time in seven weeks, I not only heard but had to obey the call of nature during my morning run. I stepped approximately one foot off the trail and then realized that I was no longer standing on proven ground. It sure makes you appreciate Canada when you consider that due to the risks of mines here, one misstep like this could be life threatening.

There seems to be an increasing number of stray dogs in the vicinity of our camp despite our efforts to live-trap and haul them away. It doesn't help that the guards at the gate often feed and pet this collection of pathetic looking mongrels. I am starting to wonder if the Bosnian we hired to take the dogs away during the day is secretly trucking them back into the area at night – that would be a very clever way to ensure he remains employed. This sounds a lot like something my old friend Dick Hartnett might have thought of as an income-generating scheme. Some of our troops have had dogs attack them and a few have been bitten. I was lunged at by a beast with bared fangs this morning, and it wasn't even the RSM (Regimental Sergeant Major). Fortunately for me, I was able to intimidate the angry dog, and he backed off, thinking a bite from me might be more dangerous than a bite from him.

Clinically, we have been quite busy the last two days. One of the local carpenters got his left thumb caught in a radial arm saw which left the tip of his thumb resembling raw hamburger meat. I did the best I could to put it back together, and now I have to trust that Mother Nature will work her healing miracles. We also had two young Canadian women show up at the front gate requesting treatment from our medical staff. We agreed to see them, and they were escorted to the UMS. Upon their arrival, one of the medical assistants took me aside to tell me that he would do me a big favour and see both patients. Although I suspected his interest in reducing my workload was not entirely unselfish, I agreed to back off. What we didn't realize was that as we were having this discussion, the senior medical assistant snuck in from behind and stole the patients right out from under our noses. I don't think I have seen him move that quickly the entire time we have been in theatre.

The ASC has been undergoing a significant facelift over the last few days. The operating room now has wider doors to accommodate patients and equipment. Walls have been moved and removed. Fume extraction systems have been installed and every major piece of equipment is being tested to ensure it is working properly. The CO may not recognize the place when she returns from her leave.

---

29 August 1998

The mail will be delivered to our camp tonight, and the longer people are here, the more they seem to look forward to getting something from the people who care about them. It doesn't matter what the mail is – what matters is that it provides a link to the reality you long to be part of once again. Since I am very visually oriented, I find receiving photographs to be particularly meaningful.

I realized this morning that the Pembroke soccer tournament began today, and I must admit that I felt a huge twinge of longing in my heart. This special event has become an annual community adventure, and I dearly wish I could have shared in the fun and games with all the folks from Russell. My one consolation is that I know there will always be next year.

The war council met in Drvar this afternoon, but I was unable to attend because I am required in camp to provide medical coverage. I can't say that I really minded, as it gave me the opportunity to sleep in a little and enjoy a quieter day. These briefings are starting to become very routine, and the Three Amigos are losing their motivation to attend them. This is especially true when you realize how little meaningful input you have to contribute at most briefings.

People are starting to get tired of being on the go seven days a week, and when there is possible downtime, the Army manages to find pointless little tasks to fill up every hour of the day. It almost seems like they are worried that if the troops are given any time to think, they might begin to question some of the dumb rules they have to live by.

Speaking of rules, our JAG informed us that the document of regulations generated to control this operation is now thicker than the Criminal Code of Canada, and he wasn't joking. There are rules governing drinking, fraternization, relationships with non-Canadian personnel, welfare, telephones, arcade machines, ad infinitum.

I have a picture of our new kitten Skye Blue stuck to my computer. It sure would be fun to play with her for a few minutes. She won't really be a kitten when I finally get to meet her, but I hope that we will still be able to bond.

I read an interesting article this evening. It appears that a cemetery worker in Germany recently heard music coming from Beethoven's tomb. Scientists were brought in to investigate, and after considerable study, they discovered that the sound was Beethoven's 5th symphony being played backwards. Curious as to the origin of the music, permission was obtained to exhume the grave. When they finally opened his grave, their questions were indeed answered, as they discovered Beethoven's body was decomposing! Hooah!

-----

30 August 1998

It was a very sad day for our troops, as the Canadian contingent lost its first soldier tonight. Apparently, a patrol consisting of four Cougars (armoured vehicles) was travelling along a winding mountainous road when the second vehicle suddenly veered right and plunged 150 metres down a cliff. The driver was thrown from the vehicle and sustained severe head and abdominal injuries. The other two soldiers remained in the vehicle and miraculously survived with relatively minor injuries. The trailing crew of soldiers contacted the medical team from Zgon, and an ambulance was dispatched and an airevac initiated. The medical team went down into the ravine over unproven ground and stabilized the seriously injured patient. Then they had to lift him safely back up the 150-metre embankment. He was conscious when they first reached him, but he slipped into unconsciousness during the journey back to base and went into cardiac arrest just as they arrived. The British helicopter with an anaesthetist on board had just arrived, and they ran a thirty-minute

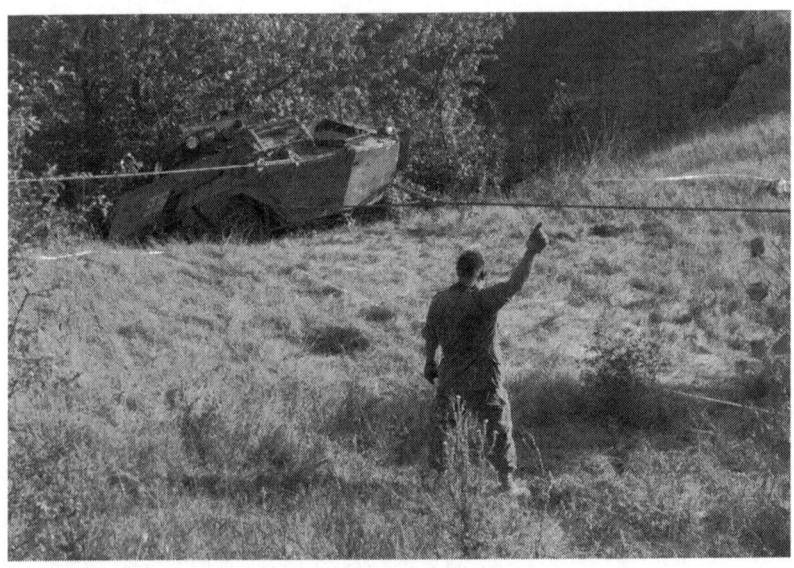

Extracting the badly damaged Cougar vehicle after it went over the cliff was complicated, especially with the potential for land mines in the area.

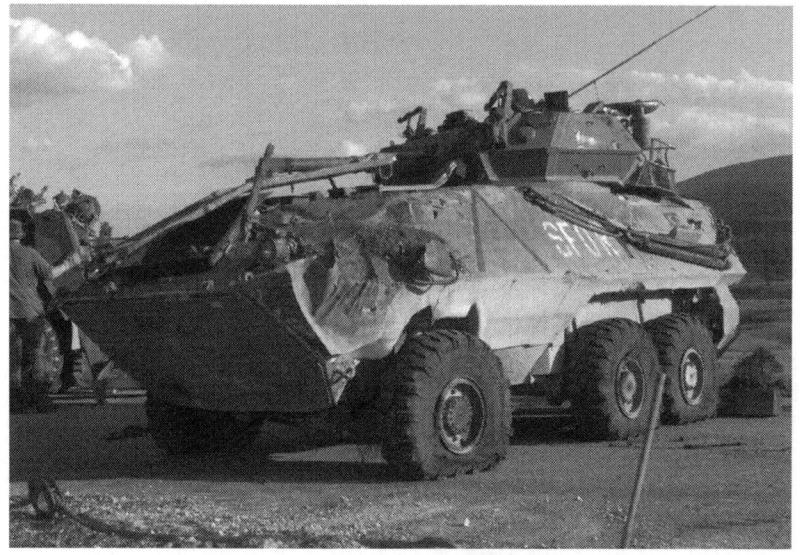

**The badly damaged remains of the Cougar vehicle when it was
finally returned to the road.**

resuscitation but were unable to revive him. Tragically, he was pronounced dead at 2230hrs. The deceased was a young man with a wife
and no children. As I considered this tragic loss, I couldn't help wondering how hard it will be for his wife to accept that someone she loves could
have died so very far away from home trying to keep peace in a country
which has gone to great lengths to destroy itself. When you look at it
closely, it hardly seems worthy of such a sacrifice.

When someone dies in a theatre of operation, an enormous number of actions immediately kick into motion to protect the remains,
inform the next of kin, get the deceased home for a funeral and protect the personnel who may have been psychologically traumatized by
the death. The first thing that happens is a complete communications

lockdown to prevent calls back home which could inadvertently get back to the next of kin and cause considerable embarrassment and pain. Before the CAF started using these communication lockdowns, wives would sometimes learn through the rumour mill that their husbands were dead only to find out that they hadn't even been injured.

The deceased was delivered to the ASC at approximately 0330hrs, and a team of medical people prepared the body to be placed in the morgue. We had a large number of volunteers who were willing to stay up and assist with whatever was necessary. The unit managed to locate his wife in his hometown. She took the news of his death very hard and was ultimately admitted to the hospital for sedation. I can't begin to think how painful it would be to have a stranger knock on my door and inform me that my spouse won't be coming home alive. Please Lord, help this young man's family. I have a feeling that tomorrow will be a very long day.

---

31 August 1998

It has been relatively quiet here for the last few weeks, but in the last twenty-four hours, we have had a shoulder dislocation that required heavy sedation to reduce, a tragic accident resulting in the death of a Canadian soldier, and a Czech soldier with acute appendicitis who required surgery in our facility. I was so swamped by the administrative preparations for returning our deceased soldier home that the surgical team didn't even bother to call me in to assist with the appendectomy. I am very disappointed at having missed out on this opportunity to be involved in some field surgery. Maybe I'll get another chance before it is time to head back home.

Today was a never-ending storm of phone calls about autopsies, morticians, flights, equipment, embalming, travel plans, updates, death certificates, caskets, hearses, escorts and money. The Canadian Armed Forces are doing their very best to treat the deceased and his family with the utmost respect, and I am truly impressed at how quickly they have reacted to this tragedy. Some of the administrative staff have been working round the clock to ensure that all the details are taken care of. The Canadian Armed Forces will be flying a mortician in from Toronto tomorrow morning. The embalming will occur Wednesday morning, and the deceased will depart Zagreb late Thursday afternoon. There are a number of memorial services planned for every military unit that the deceased body will pass through. I am very tired, and I am worried that I may have forgotten to do something. I have been asked to accompany the body until it is safely aboard the Hercules aircraft. In addition, the deceased's remains will have an escort from the Battle Group from the time he leaves Coralici until he is returned to his grieving family. This is a gesture of respect, a very important issue for the Army.

I have finally figured out the source of the emptiness that I feel here in theatre. I am truly incomplete without my family, and it is not something that keeping busy twenty-four hours a day can resolve. All this work does help to distract me, but in the end, I return to the same basic truth: I am nothing without my family. Guardian angels of mine, please keep a close watch over them. Amen.

DIARY OF A DEPLOYED DOC

September 1998

1 September 1998

The excitement here never ends. This morning, I was supposed to accompany the remains of our departed soldier to Zagreb, but this plan was changed at the last minute because we don't have enough general duty medical officers around to provide adequate coverage to the Battle Group. Our soldier's body made it safely to Zagreb where it will be stored in the Forensic Science Centre overnight. Tomorrow, the mortician from Toronto will conduct the embalming and the deceased will be loaded into a Hercules aircraft and flown back to his family. May he forever rest in peace.

NDHQ left me a message indicating that the Surgeon General would like to come and visit in six days' time. I spent a great deal of time preparing a note to explain to the staff officers at headquarters why this was a very bad idea, only to find out that they had in fact given me the wrong date, and he would be arriving in thirty-six days.

The teaching session today on the examination of the back was almost cancelled because the lecturer was unexpectedly called away. I volunteered to give the talk in his place and spent two hours teaching the medical staff. Just to sweeten things up even more, I was informed that the Division Surgeon was popping in for an unanticipated visit, and he managed to arrive one hour late. We ended up giving him and his guests a tour and having lunch with them. As if this wasn't enough, 5th Corps' ammunition site (5th Corps was one of the seven corps of the Bosnian army) ammunition site located twenty kilometres from Coralici had a massive explosion today, and many civilians were instantly killed or badly injured. Apparently, our weapons inspection teams have been predicting this for a long time. In their words, "The place was a disaster waiting to happen." We deployed our quick response team as well as an ambulance crew and had the surgical team on standby for three hours. In the end, we did not receive any casualties. The older staff were relieved to hear this, and the younger staff were very disappointed because they were hoping to see some action.

I found out today that the people who work in the cement factory adjacent to us get paid only thirty Deutsche Marks per month – this is the equivalent of about twenty-five Canadian dollars or thirty-five cents in American currency. The employers get away with grossly underpaying their staff by claiming that times are tough and they cannot afford to pay them more. The workers are trapped in that they cannot afford to give up their job because if the economy ever improves and they have been loyal to the company, they will continue to have a job. It sounds like another trick by the local mafia to get richer while the poor continue to be taken advantage of.

---

2 September 1998

An engineer with the local demining team informed me that the recent ammunition dump explosion was triggered by an individual trying to put a 122mm mortar shell back into a damaged container. When the round wouldn't fit properly, he apparently slammed the lid down on top of the round and this activated the firing mechanism. The round detonated instantly, disintegrating him and two of his co-workers. The explosion then triggered a sympathetic reaction that detonated all the ammunition in the vicinity. In the end, a number of buildings were completely levelled, and many people were burned and injured from flying shrapnel. Apparently, the engineers hated going to inspect this particular site because the explosives were deteriorating and becoming increasingly unstable. Our on-site medical personnel described the scene as resembling a fire in a box of fireworks. There were artillery rounds going off in all directions and this continued even when our engineers went into the site in their armoured vehicles. The Bihac hospital received all the casualties, and the surgeon there described the scene as nothing new for them having just survived a brutal war.

Today I finally finished a set of emergency phone numbers for all the major units and medical facilities within eight hours of our camp. This took a great deal of work as everyone speaks different languages, and there are six different phone systems. I had just returned from making copies for everyone when I got an e-mail indicating that the prefix for one of the telephone systems had changed. The timing of this event was just too coincidental for me to believe that the Army didn't plan this change just to try and drive me nuts. I've got news for them – I have been here for a long time now, and I don't plan on losing my mind any time soon.

One of the issues that the contingent leadership is continuously emphasizing in theatre is "mine awareness." With this in mind, I have started referring to the alcohol consumption policy as the "wine awareness" program.

This evening, as we were doing our fitness walk, my walkie-talkie went off, but the transmission was undecipherable. Our surgeon quickly grabbed the device from me and announced with a straight face that the secret to obtaining clear transmissions was all in how you handle your antenna. I had to bite my lip to keep from jumping on that line. When we finally received a clear transmission, we were told there was a patient being sent to us with either appendicitis or a cardiac problem. This is an unusual differential diagnosis as these two conditions present very differently. When we arrived and asked how our appendix patient was doing, we were informed that his appendix was not the problem – he was having "a panic attack." So much for our old ears. Maybe I can get a pension for being deaf and dumb – I certainly won't have any trouble proving the dumb part.

3 September 1998

Our deceased soldier was flown home in a Hercules aircraft yesterday and should have landed in Canada today. Compounding the obvious tragedy of his death, I just discovered that he was scheduled to fly home on leave, on the very day his remains were delivered to his loved ones in a coffin draped in the Canadian flag. At the repatriation ceremony, Col Natynczyk summed it up best by saying that the deceased was here to help bring peace to Bosnia – now may he rest in peace. His embalming was done yesterday morning, and our hospital warrant officer was the attending medical representative. She described the forensic institute as a veritable "little shop of horrors." There were bodies in various states of decomposition lying scattered everywhere throughout the non-refrigerated rooms. The smell was overpowering and the non-medical personnel that accompanied her were nearly overwhelmed by the entire affair.

With Captain Edora away, I am finding it nearly impossible to get anything done because of the increased demands on my time. While this is helping time go by faster, it is also frustrating.

This morning, I felt very good and was running quite well until I felt a small nagging ache in the middle of my right hamstring muscle. The discomfort continued to intensify until I backed off a little and jogged for the remainder of my workout. My hamstring has felt tight ever since. Ordinarily, this would not have been a big deal for me, but the Terry Fox ten-kilometre run will be held here in three days, and I want to be able to perform well. I will keep my fingers crossed that the great God of healing will shine her countenance upon me.

I decided to try a new strategy to get a better file cabinet for my office. I approached the Camp Commandant indicating that I keep classified files and need to be able to lock them up at night. He agreed that this was an important security issue, and when I showed him the piece of trash I currently have, I thought for certain he would recognize that it was clearly on its last legs and then issue me a nicer one. No way. The metal techs took that pathetic hunk of junk away and somehow managed to weld a security bar onto it. From the looks of things, the security bar is worth more than the cabinet. I will find some passive-aggressive way to seek my revenge.

4 September 1998

This is supposed to be the start of the big weekend before the elections. Everyone is anticipating trouble and praying that it will not occur. The DNZ party is having a rally in VK, and intelligence sources expect some thirty thousand people to attend. The DNZ is a Croatian-backed organization, and the Croatians want to acquire this part of Bosnia. The SDA represents the Bosniak element of the population, and our intelligence personnel have discovered that the SDA supporters who live in the VK area are sending their families away for the weekend. This is not a good sign. The Battle Group is going to provide a "robust" presence for this rally and they will be supported by one hundred Carabinieri – the Italian riot control police. If things do get out of hand, we are hoping that Ottawa will allow our soldiers to use pepper spray to defend themselves. You would think that allowing Canadian soldiers to defend themselves while keeping the peace in a foreign nation would be a pretty simple issue. Heaven forbid the pepper spray causes some discomfort to someone who is attacking our soldiers. I would like to put some of our politicians' children on the front line and then see what level of force they would allow them to use to defend themselves. Our country needs some senior leaders who have the brass marbles to stand up and support our soldiers at the vanguard. I will be going up to VK tomorrow morning so that we have a physician present in this potential hot spot. We have a plan for medical evacuation to our hospital if required – I hope things do not deteriorate to this point.

My other two amigos left for their R&R last night, and things have been very quiet without them. As the JAG was preparing to leave, I asked his paralegal to give him a package that I put together for his journey. When she handed him the box of 144 Trojan condoms, he only smiled and asked if this was all I could manage to spare. I am assuming he was disappointed that his weekend exploits would be cut short by an insufficient supply of protective equipment. He and the PsychO have been looking pretty tired, but he has clearly not lost his sense of humour. I imagine a few days away from Stalag Coralici will do them both a world of good. I think in three weeks I will be very ready for a break from all the long hours I am working.

Good night world. Dear Lord, please continue to look after my family. Amen.

---

5 September 1998

Well today is the big day for the last round of political rallies before next weekend's elections, and the Battle Group is preparing for any eventuality. The morning O-Group (Orders Group) lasted over two hours with every unit outlining how they would try and make as large a presence as possible and what they would do in the event of trouble. The Commander also discussed the issue of the boredom that may follow the election period and referred to this period as the "dog days." He asked the leaders in the Battle Group to think of some strategies to help combat it. During the Commander's round table, one of my comments was that the medical team had come up with a strategy to help with the dog days. I told them with a straight face that we had ordered a large supply of Viagra to help keep morale "up." I then informed him that, regrettably, the shipment had been stolen this morning as it crossed the border from Croatia. I requested that everyone in the Battle Group keep their eyes open for any "hardened" criminals in the AOR. Fortunately for me, everyone thought this was funny.

This region of Bosnia was blessed with rain from the time the rallies began until the late evening. There were no major incidents during the rallies, and one cannot help but believe that the weather had a whole lot to do with this. Thank you, Lord!

This afternoon, we had our second soldier present with significant chest pain, and physiologic markers suggested he had experienced a possible heart attack. We airevaced him to the UK hospital in Sipovo and the transfer went as smoothly as possible. Unfortunately, our team is getting better at doing this type of work because of all the practice we get moving ill and injured personnel to where they can receive the level of care they need. The patient is currently doing very well.

I took the time to make a stand for my printer out of scrap wood the carpentry shop throws out. It turned out pretty good and is a welcomed addition to my lowly office space. I guarantee that my office will be a great deal more professional looking before I depart.

The ASC had a "junk food party" this evening in their stand-easy tent. This tent is a place where the medical staff can relax and let their hair down. Despite the floor being flooded from the heavy rains, a good time was had by all. Everything served was hot and spicy, and I know my guts will be churning tomorrow. I really enjoy being with the medical staff here, they are professional when they need to be but can have fun when they want to. I think this is a healthy formula for success.

---

6 September 1998

It is the end of week eight and I only have twenty more to go. Ouch! I am trying not to think that way but focus instead on dealing with the challenges each new day throws my way.

Janet sounds like she is coping well, but she is getting worried about her upcoming licensing exams. She has worked very hard – it will be nice for her to finally have a long and well-deserved break.

Today we had our Terry Fox run on the infamous heart route. They offered two times to run: at 0800hrs and at 1800hrs. I elected to run during the rainy morning because I am on call today. My right hamstring felt fine during my easy warm-up and didn't bother me until thirteen-minutes into the race when I felt the first twinge. It was tolerable until the nineteen-minute point when I experienced a very painful tug, and I knew the muscle was now torn. Although it was initially quite painful, I managed to finish the run, and to my amazement, I also managed to remain in the lead. While I should have been happy simply to finish, let alone win, I am quite disappointed because I was on my way to achieving a very fast time before my aging body gave out on me. I then got to wait for ten and a half hours to see if the next group of runners could better my time. Fortunately for me, the closest anyone came to my time was forty-five seconds slower. To celebrate my victory, I was given a 3 RCR tank top to round out my already outstanding war-zone wardrobe. You can imagine how happy the Army was that a nearly forty-four-year-old Air Force medical officer with a torn hamstring beat all their soldiers. I love it! Hooah! Hooah!

At Mass today, we found out that our application to take a trip to Medjugorje was approved. I am very excited about this opportunity to visit a place of such great religious significance, and I only hope that nothing interferes with my going in early October.

Sunday has become my room-cleaning and domestic-improvement day. The blankets we are issued are so narrow they barely cover the top of the bed, and they always fall onto the floor, leaving you freezing to death at night. To rectify this problem, I used #1 Prolene suture material to sew my two blankets together to make one giant blanket that will hopefully stay put. I will give my innovation a trial run tonight.

The Commander left for some much-needed R&R this afternoon. He has been a very busy boy, and he is likely to remain very busy for the rest of this tour.

---

7 September 1998

As I wrote the date this morning, I realized that this is the first day of my twenty-fifth year of military service. For the majority of the Battle Group that means I joined the CAF three to four years before they were born. I am sure in the eye of the troops that officially makes me older than most fossils!

Today was pretty routine until approximately 1600hrs when a patrol called in to report that two vehicles had gone off the road and ended up in an area that is known to be heavily mined. The engineers were tasked with clearing the area and extracting the vehicles. It is standard operating procedure for the BG to deploy an ambulance with the convoy of vehicles used in these taskings, and I decided to tag along and learn more about what everyone here does. I had no idea what I was getting myself into. First of all, the ten-minute journey to the site ended up taking forty minutes and landed us right on the Croatian border. The roads kept getting smaller and smaller to the point that they were narrower than our armoured ambulance. When we finally stopped at the edge of a forest, the soldiers in the lead vehicle began pulling out maps – a sure sign that we were lost. Getting lost in Canada is one thing, but being lost in an overseas minefield is a whole different matter. You can't simply turn your vehicle around and drive back, because this would involve leaving the road and risking being blown sky-high. Instead, we had to carefully back up till we got to the proper road, at which point the engineers went in and left the rest of us on standby, approximately two kilometres from the extraction site. It is quite romantic eating your box lunch on top of an armoured vehicle while enjoying a beautiful Bosnian sunset. The only thing missing was some fine wine, which we more than made up for by whining about our predicament.

As it steadily grew darker, it became increasingly obvious that something was wrong. Apparently, the tread system on one of the armoured personnel carriers was badly damaged, and the vehicle was so badly stuck that it would likely require a Chinook helicopter to extract it. Once it was decided that nothing further could be accomplished, we were told that we would be staying put for the night – an operational vehicle cannot remain unprotected overnight for fear it would be stripped to the bone by the morning. You can't imagine the joy I felt at the prospect of getting to sleep in the middle of a minefield, with no sleeping bag, no blanket, no wash kit and only meals ready to eat (MRE) ration packs for food.

To my utter amazement, the engineers were crazy enough to continue working in the forest long after it was dark. Not only were they at risk of being bitten by the poisonous snakes that live in the area, but they were also very much at risk of being killed or badly injured by a land mine. Headquarters finally convinced them to stop all work, bed down in their vehicles and start again in the daylight.

The medical team and the military police finally got to leave five hours after we arrived, and while this experience was educational, I can't say I enjoyed watching our troops put themselves in unnecessary danger. I hope they are OK throughout the evening. Will I ever learn how to avoid getting myself into potentially dangerous situations? I seriously doubt it!

---

8 September 1998

This is the second day in a row that I have gone to the gate at 0610hrs and found no one to train with. I normally enjoy running by myself, but in theatre, the rules are such that I cannot leave the camp without a partner. This is very frustrating for me. I really don't care if the entire contingent sleeps in while I train, but when their sleeping in doesn't allow me to train – that is a whole different kettle of fish. I ended up walking inside the camp for twenty-five minutes until I ran into some folks going out the gate and asked if I could join them.

Today was one of those miraculous days when you manage to get a bunch of little pain-in-the-butt things done. Everyone on the medical staff had a great laugh at dumb ole Dr. Darrell being stupid enough to go out yesterday with the engineers on a vehicle extraction – they all knew what I was getting myself into before I left. It would have been nice if they had at the very least given me some kind of warning. It rained all afternoon long. Our ambulance had to go back out to the vehicle extraction site, and the crew came by to see if I was still interested in coming out with them, only to be surprised when I graciously declined their generous offer. The crew told me that today's trip was even more treacherous than yesterday's because all the dirt paths were now extremely muddy. Wonderful! At this morning's intelligence briefing we were informed that the stranded vehicles were in an area that contained no less than seventeen different minefields. This left me with a warm fuzzy feeling that is difficult to put into words.

As part of our public health program, anyone who tests positive for a sexually transmitted disease is interviewed to determine who they have recently had sexual contact with. One of the men who recently tested positive for gonorrhea identified a woman from our camp with whom he claims to have had unprotected sex. This soldier is married and has absolutely nothing to gain by identifying a contact. This afternoon, I had one of our staff contact this woman and arrange for me to meet with her late in the afternoon. This is a very awkward topic, and after I gently introduced the reason for seeing her, she informed me that nothing like that ever happened. I wasn't sure if she was denying involvement because she feared disciplinary consequences, so I took my time and assured her that no disciplinary action would occur. She emphatically maintained that nothing had occurred. I then explained the reasons we bring people in for these kinds of situations, emphasizing the long-term health and fertility consequences of failing to treat such problems. Still, she continued to deny any involvement. This was embarrassing for both of us. Eventually, I contacted the home unit to recheck the soldier's story. Once again, despite having a great deal to lose by raising the issue, he stated that he had had sexual relations with the woman I interviewed. I am not entirely certain what is going on here, but I bet we haven't heard the final chapter of this story.

Thank you, Lord, for blessing me with a wonderful set of parents. May everyone in the world be so very fortunate.

---

9 September 1998

This is the second day in a row that I have been able to get a great deal done, and if this keeps up, I may eventually find myself well-organized. Heaven forbid this should ever happen. The saga of the vehicles stuck in the minefields just keeps getting scarier and scarier. This morning, I learned that the crew of the stranded vehicle had wandered two kilometres off proven trails when they got stuck. This means that when our ambulance went in for them on Monday night, we were also travelling on uncleared trails through a heavily mined area. The crew had to spend three days with the vehicle until it was finally rescued, because the BG could not leave it unattended. Rumour has it that the crew commander will be pulling shoe leather out of his rear end for a long time after the Army is through with him.

Today, I saw an interesting case of a young man with an enlarging right breast. I first met him in the minefield when he came over to our ambulance at night and asked me to examine him. Can you imagine? There we were stuck in a minefield in the middle of nowhere with absolutely no ambient light. It was so dark it was difficult to see your hand in front of your face, and this young man thought that since neither of us was doing anything useful at the moment, it was the perfect time to squeeze in a medical consultation. Initially, he was just a voice calling out in the black wilderness, "Doc, I think I am growing a boob." He did have a rather large right breast, and I warned him that if the enlargement continued, he risked becoming quite a popular fellow in the shower room. We will be sending him off for an endocrine workup, and he may elect to have the extra breast tissue surgically excised.

The CO of the ASC returns to the theatre tomorrow, and she will be in for a few surprises. Firstly, the staff have made several physical improvements to the centre. Secondly, the staff have weathered a number of real and metaphorical storms in her absence and are much more battle-hardened than they were before her departure. I hope that she finds the transition back into the saddle relatively smooth.

I was unable to run again today as my hamstring continues to be too tender to subject it to any real stress. Things have cooled off quite a bit around here, and I am now wearing Lycra tights to train. I haven't seen any other males wearing Lycra, and I have a funny feeling that in this macho Army environment it's unlikely I ever will. Wait till they get a look at some of my more colourful running stuff.

---

10 September 1998

The Camp Sergeant Major has started a new tradition of broadcasting the national anthem at 0800hrs every morning. When the broadcast starts everyone must stop whatever he or she is doing and come to attention. This is usually most comical during breakfast when everyone in the dining hall has to drop whatever they are chewing on and snap to the proper position of "AH-TEN-SHUN!"

The intelligence folks informed us that someone installed a bomb-like device in the toilet of an abandoned home that our troops were operating out of. The device was eventually shown to be a fake, but not before this became forever labelled the "shitter bomb" incident. A few times when I've been in the bathroom, my wife has expressed grave concerns that a bomb may have exploded while I was taking care of business.

This evening on our way to play soccer, I tried to come to the defence of one of my teammates who was being accused of not training frequently enough. I mentioned that, to his credit, I do see him running the trails every now and then and that I had even seen him pumping steel in the gym. The misconception that I had come to his aid lasted as long as it took one of the lads to ask, "And what platoon does Steel work in?" If these guys were as fast on their feet as they were with their wit, our soccer team would be unbeatable.

As it turns out, one of my teammates happened to be the driver of the tube-launched, optically-tracked, wire-guided (TOW) missile launcher that got stuck in the minefield. He tells me that they were lucky that their vehicle hit a tree stump and had several of its wheels knocked off because that is what ultimately brought them to a stop. If their vehicle hadn't stopped, it almost certainly would have fallen into a ravine where it probably would have rolled over and killed several of them. This young man is the proud father of a three-and-a-half-month-old baby boy, and we narrowly escaped sending him home in a body bag or crippled for life. To make matters worse, the crew commander knew that they were in mine territory and that their vehicle was definitively no longer in a cleared area. Despite knowing this, he allowed his troops to get out of their vehicle and walk around. All things considered, I think the Canadian contingent is lucky we aren't sending more of our boys back home with flags draped over their coffins.

This morning, I was informed that the bacterial counts in the water supply of two of our camps – Coralici and VK – exceed the acceptable Canadian standards. We regularly test the water available in our camps to ensure that it meets acceptable public health standards. To protect the troops, we will have to stop using the tap water for drinking, brushing teeth, cooking, and washing dishes until the source of contamination is found. Oh, this sounds like it's going to be a real gong show!

---

11 September 1998

It may not be December, but it sure felt like Christmas today. The CO of the ASC returned from her three-week leave bearing gifts from my mother and father. It was great to open packages and find my favourite candies wrapped up in T-shirts and socks. This was wonderful because I could make good use of everything they sent. The best part is that the gifts came from two of the nicest people I will ever have the privilege of knowing. The package also contained a letter indicating that my parents will be coming to visit my family during my leave period at home. This was the icing on the cake. It will be terrific to see them.

This afternoon, I had a tour of the community hospital in Velika Kladusa with the aim of determining what the Canadian contingent might be able to contribute to help the staff deliver better health care to the local population. What an eye-opening experience this turned out to be. Anyone who is unhappy with the standard of medical care that they receive in Canada should have to spend some time as a patient in a facility like this. From that day forward, I guarantee they would forever hold their peace. I met with the assistant director of the hospital and told him that our intention was to establish a prioritized list of their needs. It was amazing to see that in every department we visited, the hospital staff lacked the materials that Canadians would consider essential to the basic provision of adequate care. They did not even have items as simple as wooden tongue depressors. Instead, they have to use metal ones that can be reused but require sterilization, which is costly and time-consuming. They have no new scalpel blades, so they are forced to sterilize the ones they have and reuse them. They need bandages, needles and antibiotics. They have no small-gauge needles to use for vaccinating children so are forced to use very large needles that hurt and scare the kids. Much of their equipment is very old or non-functional. The staff stated that during the war years, enemy soldiers would occasionally come in and take whatever they needed. Others would come and take things simply to be cruel. In the end, I had a two-page list of things they really needed. I also left with a real sense that the staff thought I was just another person in a never-ending parade of people who claim they are there to help but leave and do absolutely nothing. This will not be the case with me. Even if it is something small, I will see to it that Canada somehow makes a contribution – and as you will see, I kept that promise!

Our interpreter left the hospital unhappy after seeing how the priorities of the current government are so obviously useless. While there is little or no money available for education and medical care, the government is somehow building enormous mosques in virtually every community. The common belief is that the government will continue to ignore the schools and medical centres, hoping that the do-gooders from the West will eventually come to their rescue. What a messed-up world we live in.

---

12 September 1998

This was the first day of voting in the much-anticipated elections in this country. For the past week, things have been so quiet it is almost scary in the AOR. Once again Mother Nature has chosen to pour rain on this area of the world for the entire day. This will hopefully allow cooler heads to prevail.

I am tired as this has been a demanding day. In fact, I am probably tired because this has been a pretty busy week. Each of the Three Amigos is becoming less and less tolerant of the incessant need to have pointless meetings. We are starting to question the usefulness of these meaningless events and have decided that if we feel our presence will not provide any added value, then we will not be attending. This may piss off a few folks but that is just too bad. If we don't do this, the Army will run us into the ground and keep on marching.

I got a care package from my girlfriend Janny B this evening. It was a grab bag of handy items including three Victoria's Secret catalogues. I am not sure what the intention behind providing these magazines was, but I am going to assume that Janet is hinting that she would like some of the outfits for Christmas. Hooah! The package also included a photograph of Skye sleeping on top of Baby. I hardly recognize Baby – she has grown so much since I have been away. I hope that Skye doesn't get too big before we finally get to meet face to face.

I spent much of today trying to be sure that the contingent has a good grip on the issue of providing safe water to our troops in both VK and Coralici. As the day concludes, I feel confident that things are well taken care of from a preventive medicine perspective. Now all we have to do is hope that the engineers don't take too long to come up with a viable long-term solution.

I talked to Nathan this evening. He had the chance to see Lawrence Gowan perform a concert in Russell and said that it was awesome. He also told me that Gowan was part of the entertainment tour to Bosnia last year. I would have given my left nut to see that show. I have had a loooooong day, so I think I will phone my loved ones and then hit the old fart sack.

13 September 1998

Today was the last day of voting in this year's elections, and consistent with God's plan, it has once again rained all day. We have been here for over nine weeks now, and it has only rained all day long on three occasions, and all three of these occasions were critical for the elections. You can call that a coincidence if you want, but I choose to see it as divine intervention.

Yesterday, I put my foot down three times, and to my surprise this morning my foot was still attached to my body. In the first instance, I informed the Contingent Commander that the medical team had done all it could to deal with the water contamination problem and that it was now up to the engineers to come up with the answers. This morning, I received an e-mail informing me that the Commander concurred and had informed the engineers to get on with it. In the second case, I told one of the officers in the National Command Element that I would not attend a meeting they expected me to be at because I had nothing to add and had other more pressing priorities. The Commander phoned to indicate that he understood completely and that it was fine. In the last instance, I informed the Battle Group Commander that I was willing to testify before the Board of Inquiry on the death of their soldier but that I could not commit to the nine hours that the trip would require. I also informed him that I had explained this to the board members and given them some alternative solutions, but I was getting very tired of having to repeat myself. The CO of the Battle Group informed me this morning that the situation had been taken care of and the board would accept one of the solutions I had proposed. Our PsychO likens these Army turf wars to being stuck in a cold cave with only one blanket to keep you warm. Everyone would like to steal your blanket to make themselves even more comfortable, so you must be ever vigilant to ensure it never happens. It also helps if you growl and snap every now and then just to discourage people from even thinking about coming in your direction. Unfortunately, this seems to be the way the world truly works around here.

I recently discovered that everyone in the Battle Group has been randomly assigned a number from 1 to 1006, called a "ZAP number." This number allows for the communication of sensitive information across unsecured lines without personally identifying an individual. For example, you can inform the CO that the soldier with ZAP #139 has been seriously injured and only those people with access to the ZAP number lists will be able to identify who is being talked about.

I am starting to get nervous because Janet seems to be spending money on a whole lot of things lately: house painting, a car paint job and a new dishwasher, to name but a few. I think I would prefer having her in school full-time because then she would be far too busy and tired to come up with ideas on how to drain our bank account. Janet writes six hours of licensing exams tomorrow and I pray, Lord, that you help her to relax enough to show them how much she knows.

14 September 1998

The Joint Staff (J Staff) arrived from National Defence Headquarters today and to everyone's considerable consternation announced that they were here to help. Many of us who are longer in the tooth have heard that line more than a few times in our careers. I may have even said it once or twice myself.

We were going to meet with J1 Med (Joint Staff medical officer) tomorrow, but to our surprise, he contacted us and announced that he had a great deal to discuss, so he was coming up to meet with us this evening. The bottom line was that we spent until nearly 2300hrs going over a variety of contentious theatre of operations issues. By way of introduction, J1 Med outlined his role in relation to us and the rest of the military. What scares me is that I have worked at NDHQ for over six years, but things have recently changed so much that I no longer have any idea what most of the acronyms mean, who does what, or who I should be calling. Sometimes I wonder if the Department of National Defence's (DND's) secret organizational objective is to keep us all so busy trying to keep up with organizational changes that we are incapable of recommending any real changes.

This morning, I had the pleasure of running with the CO, the Deputy Commanding Officer (DCO) and the RSM. Towards the end of the workout, the RSM asked me if I ran throughout the winter. I replied that I did and very seldom had trouble on slippery surfaces because I am so sure-footed. Less than a minute later we encountered a muddy hillside, and I slipped and fell into a ditch full of rusty barbed wire. Cut and bleeding, I finished the run, and to the RSM's credit, he was too much of a gentleman to remind me of how "sure-footed" I looked during my fall. I mentioned this to him some time later and we enjoyed a good laugh together.

During the same workout, we saw an elderly farmer dragging a ram home after it had wandered off. Well, this ram wanted nothing to do with returning home and would plant its feet firmly on the ground every time the farmer gave it a tug. The two stood there in an absolute standoff until the old man kicked the ram square in the head and continued dragging the uncooperative creature home. The farmer must have worked his butt off because we found tracks over four hundred metres in length clearly indicating some hoofed creature was sliding forward involuntarily rather than walking. Near the conclusion of the workout, the CO drew our attention to something on our left. We all turned to see what was going on, and as we did so, the CO sprinted to glory, passing through the gates first – a trick I had used on him and the boys earlier this month. Who says you can't teach the Army anything?

15 September 1998

There is nothing like being in meetings from 0900hrs until 2230hrs to make a person question their reasons for continuing to live. Not only was my rear end numb, but I could feel my already poorly functioning brain turning into pudding. While we did cover a great deal of important material, there must be a more humane way to do this. To J1 Med's credit, he remained very focused and allowed every one of us to vent our spleens – even when it was obvious that we were being repetitive.

At the end of the day, I crawled back to the tin can in which I live and collapsed into bed. The big disappointment of the day was being unable to call home to congratulate Janet on having finished her nurse practitioner licensing exams. This was a moment that she has worked hard for six years to achieve, and we couldn't share it. When you miss an important moment like this, telling someone that you couldn't get an outside line just doesn't seem to cut it. I have known Janet for a very long time, and this is the hardest I have ever seen her work to accomplish something. I wish I could hug her and tell her just how wonderful I think she is.

At the end of my runs, I have been doing some weight training, and the only other folks that are normally in the gym that early in the morning are the Special Forces guys (JTF) – we refer to them as "Those of Whom We Dare Not Speak." They usually tease me about how huge I am becoming since I have taken up weight training. It doesn't help that I am constantly asking if they have noticed how gigantic I am getting. Nice of them to humour me.

This morning, I was alone with only one of these super soldiers, and he shared that serving on all these missions has a price tag, and your family is almost always left paying. He has been married for the five years he has been with the JTF, and he has been deployed overseas for well over half of that time. He and his wife bought a boat this spring and planned a summer vacation together, only to have their plans disrupted when he was given two-weeks' notice to deploy to Bosnia. He has been here for many months now and told me he is concerned that his wife is building a life without him. I could feel the pain and frustration in this young man's voice. I can't help but wonder if this is yet another in the long list of marriages that have been strained beyond the breaking point by the unending demands for our personnel to deploy to crumbling nations. I don't think the average Canadian realizes the true price that many of our dedicated soldiers are forced to pay.

---

16 September 1998

The day started out with me trapped inside the camp again because I couldn't find any running partners. After running in circles for fifteen minutes I finally saw soldiers who were leaving the gate, and I asked if I could join. Neither of them looked like runners and neither of them looked especially thrilled to have a senior officer running with them. Much to my surprise, these two lads could really motor, and I ended up doing the spade route in 36:50 which is ten seconds faster than I had ever done it. I think they may have put on a bit of a show just for me. The temperature at the time of our run was a bone-chilling 3°C.

The contingent has finally relaxed a little and is now allowing soldiers to head out on their holidays in their civilian clothing. This may be a small thing to some, but when you are over here, it's a big deal to be able to start your holidays in a relaxed frame of mind. This evening, I went to the Mess in my "Could somebody tell me why I'm here?" T-shirt. I really wasn't sure how my fashion statement would be received. As I was selecting some items from the salad bar, one of the JTF guys came up to me and said the guys had something to say to me. When I went over to their table, they weren't at all concerned about my T-shirt but rather wanted to know where I got the grotesque set of shorts I happened to be wearing. To illustrate just how bad my shorts really were, they informed me that the fashion police would have to fine me one thousand Club Z points. You know things are bad when a bunch of dirt eatin', barbwire chewin', commando-trained, hairy-knuckled, killer bastards think your fashion sense is awful. Even worse is the fact that they took time out of their busy killin' schedule to ensure I was made aware of it. At least I can brag that I am consistently out of fashion wherever I happen to be in the world. I do miss the gentle guidance of my children when they say, "We will not go anywhere with you unless you change your outfit."

While I am on the topic of clothes, one of the senior officers here had a laundry bag go missing for over a month. As it turns out, his bag had been given by mistake to a private with the same last name. When his laundry was finally returned, he found DM800 that he had forgotten was in a breast pocket. I am thinking of proposing to the Battle Group Commander that the senior officer in question be criminally charged. When the Commander asks what for, I will recommend that the charge read that he was involved in a money laundering operation. On that ba-da-ching note I will call it a night.

---

17 September 1998

The pace of life here has finally gotten to me, and today I have less energy than I would like to be functioning with. I didn't think anyone else would notice, until one of the nurses was caring enough to remind me that I needed a relaxing evening. She escorted me over to the kit shop to help me pick out a funny video that I was going to sit down and enjoy. I did as I was told, and all the laughing did me a great deal of good. My improved mood was ultimately cut short when a soldier from Zgon arrived at the hospital requiring a workup and admission. I really must remember my mission here.

This afternoon, the CCSFOR Commander and his staff met with the J Staff for their big debriefing before they returned to Ottawa. Although I was skeptical at first, I have to say that this staff inspection visit was very constructive. It certainly helped us identify what our problems are and work out some solutions. To ensure that no one misunderstood the nature of this meeting, the Commander reminded the entire group, "If I am concerned about a given issue then we all need to be concerned about it." To which we all replied, "Yes sir!" When it came to the medical issues, he made it very, very clear to everyone in the room that he would not entertain any initiative that would remove the Canadian surgical team from his contingent. For operational commanders, their medical teams are seen as an insurance policy, and Canadian soldiers feel the same way. Believe me, the medical team is fully aware that everyone is depending on us to be there for them in their moment of need. I hope that God continues to help us meet these lofty expectations.

Once again it rained for most of the day, but it wasn't so bad because we were wearing our new Gore-Tex jackets. They really are a neat piece of kit. The soldiers can function all day long in the pouring rain and never have the water reach their skin. This is just one part of the new "Clothe the Soldier" program which should see our troops get the kind of top-quality environmental clothing they need and deserve.

Once again, our surgical team was performing humanitarian surgical procedures at the Bihac hospital. The last case of the day was a thirty-year-old male who recently had his foot blown off by a land mine in the local area. Seeing someone lying there without a limb is a vivid reminder to us all that the only safe places around here are the paved roads. I hope that all of Princess Di's work to ban the use of land mines eventually results in the eradication of these horrible weapons. I pray that no one else in my family is ever exposed to this senseless form of violence.

18 September 1998

We headed off to Banja Luka in a pea-souper of a fog. Travelling in this weather is always nerve-racking because the Bosnian people are reckless enough that a trivial thing such as zero visibility doesn't deter them from speeding down the winding narrow roads. Traffic accidents appear to be one of the major risks to SFOR soldiers, and the accidents we have seen during our time here are a testament to this fact. Just the other day another Canadian vehicle slid off the road and down a slope. The crew was extraordinarily lucky that the vehicle hit a large rock and stopped, or they would have gone over a cliff, and we would likely have been sending some of them home in coffins. Late this evening, we saw two Czech army personnel who had been in a vehicle that went off the road and rolled several times. Neither was wearing a seat belt – they were lucky to get away with only one of them sustaining a fractured wrist. Unfortunately, because of the nature of the fracture the soldier will likely require a surgical repair. I tried to put things into perspective for the young soldier by telling him that he should be very thankful that he is still alive. He is twenty-two, so I doubt that these words had much of an impact, as he is likely still under the mistaken impression that he is indestructible.

For our journey to Banja Luka, we drove in a Canadian-made vehicle known as an Iltis. The Iltis is supposed to be a four-person vehicle, but I believe that in the interest of saving money, the Canadian Forces asked the company to equip them with a back seat small enough that no one over four years of age could possibly be comfortable. Someone my size has to sit with their knees shoved up into their face. To add to your travelling comfort, if it rains the water leaks in from the roof, through the windshield and up through the holes in the floor. There truly is "no life like it"! Hooah!

While in the camp at Banja Luka, I decided that I would see about getting a haircut. When I inquired if their barber was any good, they all laughed and told me that they have nicknamed him the "Ethnic Cleanser" for very good reasons. Being the adventurous type (a polite way of saying that I am really stupid), I decided to see if the Ethnic Cleanser was as bad as they built him up to be. One of the more mischievous members of the staff escorted me to the barber's shop and informed this fellow who speaks almost no English that I wanted a "No. 1" – a cut that leaves you as close to completely bald as humanly possible. I told Mr. Cleanser that I did not want a No. 1, and he nodded his acknowledgement. For the entire time I was in his chair I wasn't sure just how much hair he was going to leave me with. In the end, I was grateful to not leave his shop as bald as a cue ball, but he did cut my hair short enough that everyone I met commented that I appeared to have had my golden locks trimmed.

---

19 September 1998

I made the executive decision to sleep in till 0740hrs this morning and enjoyed every minute of it. We had the big AOR conference this afternoon with representation by units from every aspect of the contingent. There must have been fifty people crammed into this tiny little room, and everyone had to endure several hours of grandstanding by junior officers trying to be noticed. We have many big shots coming to visit in the next short while, and the only detail that wasn't discussed was how often the VIPs would be allowed to scratch their rear ends. Not only is having to endure this overly detailed planning very boring, but it is also extremely frustrating when you have a lot of other things to get done. Fortunately for me, I was scheduled to give a lecture one and a half hours into the meeting, so I was able to excuse myself and go practice some real medicine.

Our water remains unfit for human consumption, and the engineers do not feel they will find a solution anytime soon. The soldiers responsible for this type of work are formally known as Water, Fuels and Environmental Technicians. This is quite a mouthful for your average grunt, and so they are more commonly referred to as "shit techs" – a name that I like so much, I have been using it whenever I get the chance. I sure hope these guys get things straightened out before the ground freezes.

During our meeting in Banja Luka, we were introduced to the British contingent's veterinarian who is primarily responsible for their dog unit. They have two types of canines: attack dogs that are vicious and bomb-detecting dogs that have a keen sense of smell. The British affectionately refer to them as "snappy dogs" and "sniffy dogs."

Just outside the entrance to the British camp, the locals have set up little wooden stands where they sell black-market CDs for six Deutsche Marks each. That is less than five Canadian dollars for each CD, and you can get the greatest hits of just about anyone who has ever made an album. I picked up Duran Duran, Bryan Adams, Joe Satriani, Queen, Prince, Aerosmith, ABBA, Eric Clapton, Seal and Adiemus. It is wonderful to have some great tunes to listen to while I am working late in my office.

This evening, we had a surprise visit from the Canadian flight surgeon located with our squadron of CF-18 fighter jets in Aviano (northern Italy). This young man just graduated from medical training and was given two days' notice to prepare for this tasking. He is currently responsible for only 150 air crew and is living in luxury compared to Stalag Coralici. If this wasn't jammy enough, his tour will only be three months long. While I envy him in some ways, I know he will not come out of his deployment having learned nearly as much as I will.

---

20 September 1998

Tis the end of week ten and it has rained the entire day. This sure puts a damper on things during the one day that people around here try to relax a little. We had a replacement Anglican priest say Mass today, and it was a wonderful experience. There were nine of us participating, and there was a warmth in the room coming from more than just the space heater. I was particularly impressed at the priest's ability to relate a three-thousand-year-old scripture to the situation this area of the world is currently experiencing. I think everyone in our small congregation is looking forward to his stay with us.

I find myself missing Janet a great deal the longer I am here. The Army would consider this a sign of extreme personal weakness. She and I have been best friends for a very long time, and I miss sharing little things with her. Now that she has finished her licensing exams, she seems to be coming out of the blue funk that engulfs anyone who is totally preoccupied with trying to make it through a tough program. I only hope she doesn't rebound into a lengthy renovating and spending spree.

The Queen's School of Medicine Class of 1988 is having its tenth reunion this coming weekend, but unfortunately, I have other commitments – something to do with saving a nation from self-destruction. Since I couldn't be there in person, I took a great deal of time preparing a letter to be read to them at the dinner. It is very difficult to express in three hundred words or less what life is like here and what exactly I am doing. I hope that the next time we have a reunion I will be able to attend. Most of my classmates were so young when we were in school, it would be very interesting to see how the demands of real life have changed them.

As things settle down in the post-election period, it appears that the voters have re-elected all the hard-liners back into power. While I do not pretend to understand the politics of the region, I am told the election results represent a rejection of the international community and the Dayton Peace Accord. This likely means continuing instability in the region. I am beginning to realize this situation is quite similar to that of Quebec, in that the problem child has more to gain by remaining a problem than by settling down. In the case of Bosnia, if everything suddenly becomes peaceful, then all the international support agencies and their money will disappear, and Bosnia will be left to fend for itself. On the other hand, if every so often someone throws a grenade or burns a house down, the support agencies will stay and keep injecting massive quantities of money into the economy. This isn't a nice thought, but it is the economics of survival.

---

21 September 1998

The recce team for the next rotation arrived this morning, and it suddenly dawned on me that we have been here long enough that they are starting to train our replacements. These folks have a great deal of work to do before they come into theatre, and some of them are just coming to this realization. Our contingent is melding into a very effective team, and this gives me a real sense of accomplishment. Despite all the crap we have endured, I imagine it will be hard to say goodbye in five months' time.

It appears that everyone and their dog is coming to visit us, including media teams, the Chief of Defence Staff, the Deputy Minister, the Surgeon General, the Vice Chief of Defence Staff and a host of others. The only VIPs who aren't coming to say howdy are the Spice Girls, but I am not absolutely certain they won't make a surprise appearance. These visits actually get to be a bit of a drag because of all the pomp and circumstance that is part of each visit. Perhaps the rationale is that, since we aren't currently fighting any hostile forces, we might as well struggle to host the VIPs.

I was cut off halfway through my conversation with one of my VIPs (Janet) this morning, and unfortunately, I am not allowed to call her back to tell her what happened. It is great to hear her voice with some life back in it – her nurse practitioner program took a lot out of her.

Our AOR is starting to receive refugees from Kosovo, and this is causing friction in many areas. Bosnia has a problem with its own refugees let alone those from a neighbouring nation. In addition, the locals have very little money of their own and therefore have little to share with the folks from Kosovo. The Bosnian people are starting to focus on winterization, which involves gathering enough food to eat, getting sufficient wood to keep them warm and ensuring that they have shelter from the wind and cold. From the look of their meagre homes, a cold winter would be a very difficult ordeal. The joint task force boys were in today to discuss having intravenous catheters with saline locks installed in each of them before they go in for a "hit" as they call it. A hit refers to a mission, and in this environment, it most often involves apprehending a person wanted for war crimes. In this way, if one of them were to get badly injured, the team that gets to them first would have no trouble rapidly initiating an IV. This is an interesting idea and sure shows that they are always thinking. My only concern for these highly motivated soldiers is that if the IV catheter were to be hit hard enough, it might break and release a plastic embolus into their circulatory system. That would be a bad thing, a very bad thing!

---

22 September 1998

At the invitation of the British Divisional Liaison Officer (DLO), I had the opportunity to visit the psychiatric care centre at the Bihac hospital. Describing this experience as an eye-opener falls substantially short of the mark. I am sure anyone visiting this facility would be taken aback by what they see. To begin with, the building was originally designed to handle delinquent children and not psychiatric patients. Secondly, by Bosnian standards it can maximally accommodate seventy patients but currently houses ninety-five, so saying they are at overcapacity is a gross understatement. Employing Canadian standards, this facility would be approved to house a maximum of forty-five people. Thirdly, due to a lack of space, the physicians are forced to house neurology patients with patients who have acute and chronic psychiatric disorders. Combine all this with a total lack of money to purchase modern medications, as well as a staff of only two psychiatrists, and you have the recipe for A Nightmare on Elm Street. Out of necessity, the patients are crammed into their rooms like sardines in a can. The walls haven't been painted in thirty-five years, and the smell of urine permeates the air they breathe. Despite all of this, the patients appear to be surprisingly well cared for, especially considering their limited resources. The purpose of my visit was to see for myself the dilapidated state of the facility with an eye to convincing the Battle Group Commander to have his soldiers make the refurbishing of this centre a major project. I will see what I can do. The translator who assisted us throughout the visit truly felt that the best treatment for these "defective people" was to shoot them. Perhaps this attitude is shared by many Bosnians, and that is why this facility has been allowed to deteriorate to its current shameful state. The Battle Group ended up embracing this challenging project and made huge improvements to the facility.

Following our tour, the DLO took us out for lunch at a local restaurant. It was as nice a place to eat as you will find anywhere in the world and sits in stark contrast to the rest of the town of Bihac. It is collectively owned and operated by the "Big Four." The Big Four are the most powerful mafia figures in the local area and they control everything that happens in the Bihac region. These fellas run around the city in luxurious cars while the people they have been robbing for years have very little to call their own. When you see these situations, you realize that there are always those who profit from war, and it is always the ordinary people who pay the price. This kind of stuff leaves a bad taste in your mouth when you realize that somehow, they will find a way to profit from every good thing that foreign agencies do to make life better in war-torn Bosnia.

23 September 1998

Tonight, I left Coralici for some much-needed R&R in downtown Zagreb. I have been living in a uniform behind barbed wire for so long now that it felt a little strange to be travelling in civilian clothing. We reported to VK at 2000hrs only to be informed that we could only draw our money for the trip at 0100hrs and then leave for Zagreb at either 0300hrs or 0530hrs. Only the military could conceive of this kind of stupidity as being a great way to begin a holiday. It is these kinds of issues that leave some people wondering why they bothered going on R&R in the first place. I must admit that I am tired and a few days away from all my responsibilities will do me good.

I had no idea how large the camp at VK was until I decided to go for a walk this evening. It took me over twenty minutes to walk the perimeter of the camp, and then I was stopped by two sentries and told that walking after dark was not permitted and that I would have to go back indoors. The excuse the soldiers gave me was that they might confuse me with an intruder and I could be shot. I'll sleep well tonight knowing that anyone stupid enough to crawl through the barbed wire to try and cause trouble will be shot by these two lethally armed keeners. Hooah!

I saw my first case of malaria today in a fifty-five-year-old Ghanaian policeman working with the United Nations International Police Task Force. He had developed night sweats, had coughed up some bloody sputum and generally was not feeling well. He has had malaria before, and his blood smears show malarial organisms in some of the red blood cells. Unfortunately, our pharmacy does not carry the medications he requires, so he will need to seek them through the local pharmacy – good luck with that!

Captain Edora returned today from Zgon where he was covering for Captain Chung who was away on his three weeks of leave. It is nice to have Captain Edora back. While it will make my life simpler, I will miss having the opportunity to practise so much clinical medicine.

I was recently informed that the local Bosnian police are paid approximately DM150 per month and that the average rent for an apartment in this region is DM300 per month. It doesn't take a Nobel Prize-winning mathematician to figure out that there is a problem here. It appears that the only way the police can survive is to supplement their income by extorting money from the drivers they stop on the road. One of the major roles of the United Nations International Police Task Force is to reduce local police corruption. I would suggest that the best way to ensure police corruption is alive and well in Bosnia is to continue to pay them substantially less than they need to support their families.

I've got to go now so I can get up at O dark thirty tomorrow to begin enjoying my military vacation.

Here is a little something that every Canadian citizen should have to read at least once in their lifetime:

It is the soldier, not the reporter,

who has given us freedom of the press.

It is the soldier, not the poet,

who has given us freedom of speech.

It is the soldier, not the campus organizer,

who has given us the freedom to demonstrate.

It is the soldier, not the lawyer,

who has given us the right to a fair trial.

It is the soldier who salutes the flag,

who serves under the flag

and whose coffin is draped by the flag

who allows the protester

to burn the flag.

(Included with permission from the author.)
Copyright © 1970, 2010 by Charles M. Province (Retired US Army)

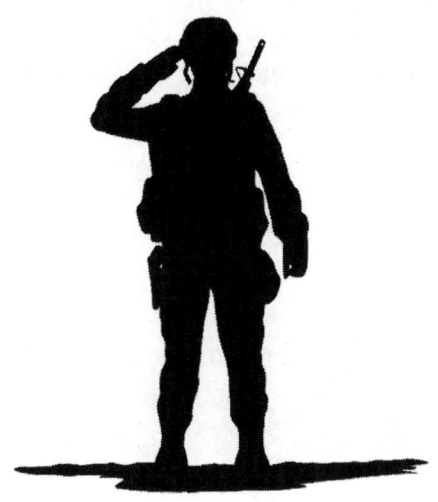

24 September 1998

Today is my first non-working day in eleven weeks, and it feels oddly like I am being let out on a weekend pass from prison. Last night I learned how to set up an army issue cot and even managed to have a good night's sleep. This may have more to do with the fact that I elected to sleep in the physician's office than it did with the inherent comfort of the cot. I chose to sleep in the office because the only other option was to sleep in the transient quarters with everyone else and the guarantee of substantial amounts of noise. From the comments this morning, it sounds like I made the right choice.

We awoke at 0500hrs to get on the bus taking us to Zagreb, from where we would all go our separate ways. When we arrived in Zagreb, I discovered there were only three of us that were staying there, which suited me fine because this significantly reduced the chances of me having to babysit young soldiers who tend to get into trouble on these trips. WO Bergdahl and I were dropped off at the train station, and despite my best efforts to get us hopelessly lost, WO Bergdahl somehow managed to find our hotel. We were booked into the Hotel Intercontinental – a five-star facility that has absolutely nothing in common with Stalag Coralici. Unfortunately, I think I am more comfortable with barbed wire and gravel than I am with door attendants and marble. This place is costing us CAN$95 per night on a special SFOR rate. The regular fee is CAN$400 per night and a can of pop is $5 – which is painful enough to say let alone reach into your wallet to pay. What is nice about the Intercontinental is that it is quiet even though it is located right downtown.

Once I got settled, I went for a great run in the forest located immediately behind the main street downtown. Following that, WO Bergdahl and I headed off to explore the downtown core. The first thing that struck us was how anyone could afford to live here especially given how poorly the local people are paid for their services.

There are posters all over town announcing that the Pope will be visiting Zagreb in October to pronounce one of their long-dead Cardinals a saint. In preparation for his arrival, the city is undergoing a huge facelift. There are workers everywhere, painting fences, mowing lawns, picking up litter and repairing the streets. All this preparation is a sore point with some folks who feel that it is inappropriate to be spending millions of dollars on a one-day visit when the government claims it has no money to spend on education and health care. One theory is that the government would rather give the people strong religious support and very little education so that they can be ruled by fear and ignorance. It sounds a great deal like the Dark Ages all over again.

Zagreb is a beautiful city, and it certainly looks nothing like the cities that lie in ruins in neighbouring Bosnia.

25 September 1998

Our medical consultant, Dr. Igor Begovic, was kind enough to spend the day taking us on a tour through the downtown region. The city of Zagreb is more than one thousand years old, and so there is a great deal of ancient stuff here to be seen. The cathedral that the Pope will visit has portions that were first built in the year 1094. Internally, it is a magnificent building, but the outer aspect is being eaten away by the by-products of pollution, which are damaging many other historic sites throughout Europe. One cannot help but wonder if the decay of this great building reflects the current status of the Catholic Church here and in many other countries. Dr. Begovic also took us to a pharmacy that has been doing business at the same location for the last 643 years – I don't imagine that anyone has ever referred to these folks as a fly-by-night outfit.

Dr. Begovic's entire life was turned upside down by the war. Everything here revolves around a person's ethnicity. It is OK to be a Muslim, Serbian or Croatian, but if you are of mixed ethnicity then you are nothing. Dr. Begovic's father was Serbian, and his mother was Croatian – a union that has been the source of unending trouble for him. I asked him how anyone would be able to tell what someone's ethnic background was, given that the people of Croatia do not appear to have any obvious distinguishing characteristics. Apparently, ethnicity is so important here that no matter what you are doing, you must be able to produce papers listing the names of your parents and their ethnic origin. Sounds a lot like Hitler is alive and well and possibly living in Croatia.

Since the war, Dr. Begovic has refused to work as a physician within the Croatian health care system because he would have to extort money from his patients to survive. Instead, he has taken a wide variety of jobs including managing a refugee camp for the UN (United Nations), working for the War Crimes Tribunal exhuming mass grave sites, and cleaning and identifying human remains. He has also worked as a truck driver and medical liaison for both the Canadian and American armed forces.

Dr. Begovic has had his life threatened by refugees he was helping and escaped only by bluffing his way out of the situation. Adding to his challenges, he came home one day to find that someone had taken over his apartment while he was at work. When he asked what was going on, a gun was put to his head, and he was told to get lost. He left but came back with two military friends armed with rocket launchers, and after getting into a fight with the thief and the corrupt local police, he finally won back his home. On the downside, he now has a police record because he refused to be taken advantage of. On another occasion, he lost his only car when it was hit by secret police officers who were drunk and driving a stolen vehicle the wrong way up a one-way street. He was bold enough to ask to have his car replaced only to be told to mind his own business. When he filed a damage claim through a lawyer, he was informed that he was being enrolled in the Croatian army and sent to the front lines. The only thing that saved him was the fact that both he and his girlfriend had previously fractured their necks in a car accident.

When I returned from a wonderful day on the town there was a message under my door to call Coralici. I knew this could not be good news because the contingent tries never to bother someone on leave unless it is extremely important. Initially, I could not get through to our headquarters because of the communication blackout put into effect whenever someone is seriously injured. When I finally did get through, I was told a twenty-three-year-old Sapper (engineer) had been electrocuted at 1400hrs while working in Camp Zgon and could not be resuscitated. So, another young Canadian life lost in uniform and another family that will undoubtedly be devastated. I also feel very sorry for Captain Chung who was still unpacking from his three weeks' leave when they brought the soldier into the UMS. Captain Chung saw the previous soldier who died three days before he left on his leave. As selfish as this may sound, this isn't going to make for much of an R&R for me, but this type of responsibility comes with the territory. Unfortunately, given our previous experience with this type of disaster, our team knows exactly what is required this time around. Lord, please be with this young man's family to help them through their pain.

----

26 September 1998

Today was a collection of phone calls and arrangements to ensure that our deceased soldier is treated with the utmost respect and is returned home to his family as soon as possible. The mortician will be flying in tomorrow, and this will mean another trip for us to the Forensic Science Centre, which would be more appropriately named the "House of Frankenstein." Dr. Begovic is very good at making the necessary arrangements and we will have the facilities, personnel and hearse when we need them.

I volunteered to remain in Zagreb to ensure that everything from a medical perspective is done properly. The Contingent Commander approved my offer. Unfortunately, this means I must accompany the deceased to the Forensic Science Centre and experience all the sights and smells that WO Bergdahl had warned us about. I am not looking forward to this at all. To help pass some of the time away, Dr. Begovic and his fiancée, Aida, took me on a trip to a small town on the border of Slovenia. It was a nice little place with some craft shops, and I managed to purchase a cute ceramic cat for my daughter Rebecca, to add to her growing collection of cat paraphernalia.

When you get to know Dr. Begovic, you can see his frustration with being trapped in a country where he is considered a nonentity.

He cannot leave Croatia at this time because both his parents are very ill, and he needs to ensure they are taken care of. He recently wrote his American medical board examinations for the third time. If he ever passes them, he would like to get accepted into a residency program in the USA and set up practice there, where no one will care that he is from a mixed ethnic background. I sincerely hope he achieves his dream.

In the evening, WO Bergdahl and I went to the cathedral and were fortunate enough to catch Saturday evening Mass. The place was packed with people who had come to celebrate the Eucharist. The atmosphere in this place of worship was so different compared to a typical Canadian Mass. It was like one of our Christmas Masses. There were four priests on the altar and the place was full of nuns in their habits. They even had novitiates in the pews. While the only word I understood was "amen," you would have had to be completely desensitized not to feel the spirituality in the air. I have always enjoyed attending religious services in foreign countries.

Although today was OK, it was tainted by the anticipation of all the things that will need to be dealt with in the next few days. I am a bit concerned because I have been having short bouts of heart palpitations since I arrived in Zagreb. I truly hope that I do not experience an episode of atrial fibrillation while I am here, as this could mark the end of my deployment and perhaps my military career.

---

27 September 1998

I slept poorly last night anticipating the embalming of our soldier scheduled for today. I went for a run in the rain hoping this would calm me down somewhat, and I think it helped a bit. The plan was to have our escort team bring the remains of the deceased to our base in Zagreb where we would meet them. Together, we would then travel to the airport to pick up the mortician and transport him to the Forensic Science Centre. When we arrived at the camp, there were two vehicles, some Canadian soldiers and a group of police at the front gate. We stopped to see what the problem was, only to discover that the Canadian soldiers were the escort team, and the vehicle that contained the remains of our soldier had just been involved in a motor vehicle accident. This may not sound like a big deal, but we are on a military base in a foreign country, with a dead body in the back of our vehicle, and a mortician who hasn't slept in forty-eight hours and who is anxious to do the embalming today. I had the administrative staff contact the military police to explain that we needed to move this body ASAP, and to our amazement, they actually listened to us.

We arrived at the Forensic Science Centre an hour late, but the staff guy was still happy to see us. You would be happy too, if you could ask for the equivalent of one month's pay under the table to allow our people to utilize a facility that isn't even yours. The embalming procedure was conducted in the United Nations facility that was built specifically to deal with the bodies exhumed from the mass graves in Bosnia. The place is full of refrigerated remains that have yet to be examined. The floor and cupboards are full of paper shopping bags with the skeletal remains of the bodies discovered throughout the war zone. This is a sad testament to man's inhumanity to man. Apparently, each of the exhumed bodies must be fluoroscoped to look for bullets to determine how they died, and the remains must be cleaned of all their flesh before they go for identification. It takes a unique person to handle this type of work – I know this would exclude me. We were in the better side of the facility, and we let the escort officer and the best friend of the deceased attend to him there.

Once the member was placed in his combat uniform, his body was draped in an engineer's flag, and we closed the coffin. We then had to take the coffin to the older part of the building, which I must admit looked like something out of a horror movie. Seven or eight bodies were lying on an old table with no refrigeration, and they would remain that way all weekend long. The place had an odour to it that is impossible to describe. To avoid traumatizing more people than necessary, I allowed only those of us who had to move the body, to go in. Before we left, I made sure the caretakers understood that only the escort or I were to have access to the body and that we took this issue very seriously – they seemed to understand.

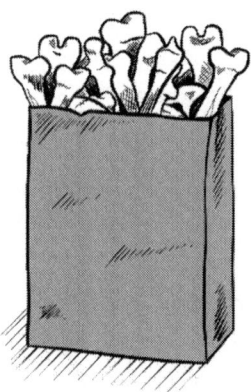

Human skeletal remains in lunch bags

The escort team was kind enough to bring up my uniform, which had been packaged up by our surgeon and anaesthetist. I was very grateful that this could be arranged. After I got my uniform on, I could feel things in pockets that I do not normally put things into. Upon further investigation, I discovered in front of the entire escort team that my colleagues had hidden condoms in everything I owned – in my combat carrying case, my briefing pads, my breast pockets and my pant pockets. They even sent me a tube of lubricating gel to enhance the quality of my stay. I will have to think of some way to seek my revenge on these devious fellows.

---

28 September 1998

I must head back to Coralici tonight, and so I had to check out of the hotel early this morning. When the cashier provided me with the bill, I whipped my wallet out of my breast pocket only to have one of the condoms my colleagues had hidden in my uniform fly through the air and land right on the counter between the two of us. We both looked at the rubber, and without saying a word, I simply placed it in my pocket and continued to pay the fellow. I think that I might have had a harder time dealing with the situation if the cashier had been of the gentler sex.

Today the remains of our deceased Canadian soldier are to be loaded onto a military aircraft and flown back to Canada. My responsibility was to ensure that his body was removed from the Forensic Science Centre and taken by hearse to the airport where the contingent had a special ceremony planned for 1300hrs. When we arrived at the Forensic Science Centre, we were informed that the usual driver and the Mercedes hearse would not be available to us for the time we required them. Instead, we were provided with a shabby-looking Citroen hearse. I took one look at this vehicle and informed our liaison person that there was no way I would dishonour one of our dead soldiers by driving him to the aircraft in what they had provided. It took thirty minutes but our Mercedes hearse and a sharply dressed driver finally appeared. At this point in time, I personally did not care what they had to do to make this happen so long as our soldier was being given the respect that his sacrifice merited.

Somehow, we managed to make it to the airport without having an accident. The departure ceremony was very moving, and on more than

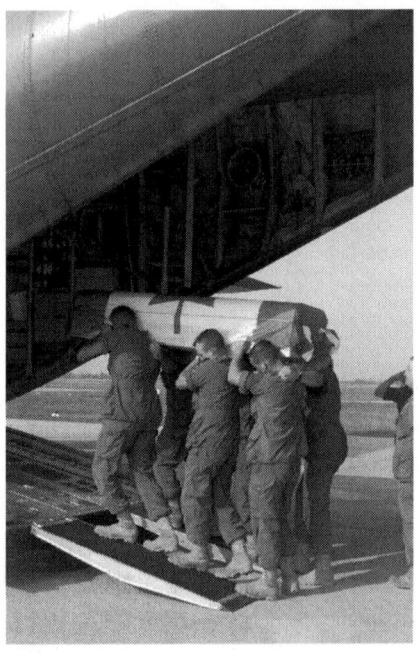

**Soldiers of the 3 RCR loading a Canadian flag-draped coffin
onto a Hercules aircraft for the long and sad trip home to
grieving family and friends.**

one occasion I displayed weakness to the Army by having a tear in my
eye. The ceremony started off with six members of his section parading
the casket draped in the Canadian flag onto the runway. Then several
scriptures were read, after which a brief homily was given. Following
this, every engineer in the contingent was given the opportunity to pay
their respects. The Contingent Commander then pinned his medal to
his coffin and said, "This young soldier came to help bring peace to this
part of the world. May he now rest in peace." The piper played a lament,
and the bugler played the "Last Post." The entire parade then accompanied the casket to the awaiting airplane and watched as our deceased

comrade was carefully loaded onto the aircraft for his long journey home to his family in Canada. When it was all over, I was impressed by the dignity and attention that was paid to commemorate this tragic loss. I will pray for his parents, as they must carry on after him, which I know I would find unimaginably difficult.

---

29 September 1998

Despite the recent tragedy to befall our contingent, the sun shone today, and life seems to be carrying on. This morning, we had the opportunity to go to the range and practice firing our 9mm pistols. Heaven help us if we are ever in a position where my shooting skills are required to keep us safe. We were each given thirty rounds to fire at close range at a relatively large target. I managed to hit the target a grand total of fourteen times, and of those fourteen hits, only three would have disabled the attacker. One of our medical assistants used to be a competitive shooter and all his rounds were within a six-inch grouping in the middle of the target's chest. While I am sure that my pathetic pistol performance caused my Indigenous ancestors to roll over in their graves, I am also hoping it convinced them that I made a wise choice to become a healer and not a hunter.

I had one of those days where everything that I touched turned to crap. It got to the point where I stopped touching things because the smell was starting to bother me. To compound my troubles, every single person in the entire camp wanted to talk to me about something important. I was tempted to touch some of them, and after they turned into a puddle of poop, I could just walk away. Could I be developing an attitude problem?

I am starting to become more involved in the humanitarian aid efforts that are so desperately needed in this shattered nation.

Unfortunately, this entire field of work is obscured by dense clouds of bureaucracy, and one must be extremely patient to be able to work one's way through it. I am slowly learning who does what, and in particular, who has the money to finance these efforts. It is evident that many people have identified specific needs, and many organizations are looking for something worthwhile to spend their money on. What they both need is someone in the middle who can bring the two groups together. This is what I hope to do because I feel this is where someone in my position can do the most good in the four remaining months of our deployment.

Today, I introduced the Battle Group to a project to help give the psychiatric facility at the Bihac hospital a much-needed facelift. I provided them with photographs from my visit and indicated that money was available for the materials that would be needed, but the people involved needed a team of trained people to do the work. In my opinion, this would be a great project for a company of soldiers to take on, and hopefully the Battle Group will accept the challenge.

Several of the churches back home in Russell are raising money to help Bosnia, and I spent the evening preparing letters for them to explain the type of work Canadian soldiers are doing. There certainly is no end to the number of things that one can do to help here.

I sure do miss my family, and it won't be long till I get to see them.

---

30 September 1998

Thirty days hath September, April, June and November. That's another month done and only twenty-one more days till I get to hug my wife and kids.

Now that Captain Edora has returned, I am getting to do a lot less hands-on medicine, and this is hard for me to handle. This morning, I was asked to start an IV on a patient who was anxious about needles, and the staff were having trouble getting the IV in place. Never fear! Dr. Darrell came flying to the rescue, and after only five tries I finally got his IV established. The patient didn't seem to mind all the poking, but it sure left me feeling professionally incompetent. I warned the young fellow not to drink anything for several days because he had so many holes in him that he might leak like a water sprinkler. I should have told him not to feel too bad because it also took me five tries to get my driver's licence.

Our helicopter landing pad was completed several weeks ago, and we now have several helicopters a day landing in our camp. It is exciting to see these technological marvels land and take off. I hope that I get an opportunity to fly in one before our tour is over. We used the pad today to have one of our soldiers taken to the German hospital near Sarajevo. We aren't sure what is wrong with him, but he is requiring a lot of pain medication, and we would like an internal medicine opinion. I hope he is OK.

The calm in the AOR seems to have dissolved in the aftermath of the elections. SDA supporters are driving around the VK area and terrorizing DNZ supporters with illegal weapons and grenades. Yesterday, a home in VK was broken into and a gunfight ensued. As usual the corrupt civilian police force is doing nothing. In response to this situation, the Battle Group has taken over and has set up roadblocks using armoured vehicles with serious firepower mounted on them. They are stopping vehicles at random to search them and the people in them. I drove to and from VK this evening, and there is a heavy military presence on the road. While this will hopefully reduce the volume of ethnically motivated intimidation we are seeing, it does put our soldiers at increased risk of violence or motor vehicle accidents.

October 1998

1 October 1998

We had the Deputy Minister of National Defence, the Deputy Chief of the Defence Staff and several other generals visiting our humble home today. They are flying all over the place using Czech and British helicopters. While this type of travel allows them to move around the AOR very quickly, it does not give them a feel for what the soldiers who drive these roads must contend with daily. The Deputy Minister of National Defence is a recently appointed civilian who has no previous experience working in DND let alone ever wearing a uniform. I do not understand why the government appoints people who have no idea what we do into senior positions like this and then wonders why things sometimes go wrong. The Battle Group put together a guard of honour for the Deputy Minister's arrival, and it was somewhat embarrassing to witness this mini-parade and realize the Deputy Minister had no idea how to stand on the podium let alone how to inspect the troops. I am sure this will change when the Deputy Minister has been in the job for a while.

We have had more bad news in that one of the soldiers who presented to us with blood in his urine has just been diagnosed with a kidney tumour and must head back to Canada for surgery. Our rotation seems to be getting more than its fair share of these kinds of serious medical problems. I hope that he does well back in Canada.

The Surgeon General, BGen Auger is coming to visit the AOR next week and I will be his aide-de-camp – which means that I get to travel all over the place with him and ensure that nothing goes wrong. I imagine if something does go wrong, I will be blamed for it and expected to fix it. This tasking involves a great deal of planning, as he will be travelling from Zagreb to Sarajevo and back again. I hope that I can organize a visit for him that will help to give him a very clear understanding of the demands involved in providing medical care in this theatre of operations.

The young soldier that I mentioned several weeks ago who was concerned about the growing distance between him and his wife informed me today that it has been a very bad week. He looked exhausted and admitted that he had slept very little in the last three nights. I suspect that yet another military marriage has dissolved in the stressful solvent of excessive deployments.

This week another medical assistant who worked amidst the horrors of the Rwandan genocide was admitted to hospital with acute suicidality. It is tragic how many of our military personnel are suffering from PTSD (post-traumatic stress disorder) as a result of the trauma they have experienced trying to keep peace in the dysfunctional world in which we live.

I forgot to mention that while WO Rose Bergdahl and I were in Zagreb, we decided to abscond with a poster of the Pope's visit. When we finally found one, I stood guard while Rose attempted to take the poster off the door of this large building. Just as she got the poster free, a nun opened the door and caught us red-handed. She reprimanded us in Croatian and then asked us to wait. We thought she was going to call the police and we would be locked away forever. Instead, she came out with a new poster, which she gave to us. We are praying that her religious order wasn't named "Our Ladies of Unrelenting Revenge."

---

2 October 1998

The highlight of my day was finding out O. J. Simpson's Internet address: slash, slash, slash, backslash, escape.

Taking care of people can be a frustrating experience at times. Today, I spent all my time coordinating the Surgeon General's visit and trying to get our soldier with the renal tumour back home as comfortably and as rapidly as possible. For the soldier being repatriated to

Canada, we were trying to use a regularly scheduled CAF flight out of Split, Croatia, but it was departing before we could get our patient transported to the airport. Trying to be creative, I asked the air medevac folks out of Winnipeg if they could simply have the flight delayed for medical reasons, and man did this ever get the ball rolling. Before I knew what was happening, the air medevac folks had escalated this event into a full-fledged medical evacuation, complete with attending nurse, medical assistant, medical assistant in training, stretcher, as well as oxygen, and IV capability. The flight schedule was completely changed, the crews were switched, and they are now going to deliver him directly to Ottawa and straight to the National Defence Medical Centre. This is outstanding service and certainly demonstrates how serious our people are about helping deployed soldiers who are ill or injured.

I had a chance to talk to the soldier this evening. It is a real pity that such a nice young man should have to contend with such a serious illness so early in his life. I ran into him as he was heading over to phone his mother and give her the bad news. Can you imagine the pain she will be going through this evening? Lord, please be there to soften the blow for her.

I was scheduled to leave on my pilgrimage to Medjugorje at 1800hrs today but unfortunately could not make it because the details for our soldier's trip home were not yet finalized. I am very disappointed, as I believe this would have been an exceptional experience. However, I am at peace with the decision to stay as I believe that getting this young man home is what God wanted me to do, and I hope that the Blessed Virgin understands why I stood her up.

I am discovering that when God wants you to do something, it just seems to happen. This evening, a young officer that I do not know came up to me and said, "Sir, I understand that you are coordinating all the medical humanitarian aid efforts?" I was about to say, "Not really," but instead elected to ask him why he was asking. He then proceeded to tell me that his father was the commander of a large, retired military members' organization and they were wondering if I could give them an itemized list of the types of things needed here in Bosnia. I told him to come and visit me tomorrow, and I would give him all the information I could. The most exciting part of this whole humanitarian effort is that it is happening largely without any help from me. The Lord does indeed work in mysterious ways!

---

3 October 1998

I slept in until 0750hrs this morning and it felt great. The BG held a brief medal parade for the young soldier who is being medically repatriated today. This is an important ceremony for everyone because it is your last chance to pay your respects to a comrade with whom you have served. I sure hope that no one in the contingent is envying him returning to Canada because I am certain he is in for a long, hard ride. Lord, please watch over this young soldier and help the people who treat him to be able to cure his problem. Amen!

Intelligence reports indicate that since the election there has been a growing level of violence perpetrated by SDA party supporters, and the violence and intimidation are being directed largely at DNZ party supporters. What is especially disturbing is the total lack of response by the civilian police force. In fact, civilian police have been identified as some of the people who are committing these acts of violence.

A member of the local police was recently caught flashing a laser pointer at our vehicles. This wasn't some sort of playful gesture – it was a deliberately dangerous act that could have blinded our driver and put everyone in the vehicle at risk of serious injury. We aren't sure if this irresponsible officer was subsequently punished or promoted but given what we have witnessed since we have been here, I would bet a month's pay he has moved up a rank or two for his bad behaviour. It is difficult to restore security to an area when the local police are a big part of the problem.

Our information propaganda personnel are working hard to send out positive messages about SFOR and what we are trying to do for Bosnia. To achieve this goal, they are using local radio station broadcasts, TV spots, personal contacts and their own widely distributed newspaper. It seems that information warfare is a big part of any mission.

The situation in Kosovo continues to heat up, and there is concern that if NATO launches an offensive, soldiers working on other NATO missions such as ours could be at increased risk for acts of retaliation. We will be at particularly high risk because of our close proximity to Kosovo and the number of Serbs in our AOR. This is all we need to make life around here more interesting.

We are now into hunting season in Bosnia, and we expect to have a hard time telling the bad guys from the legitimate hunters. Let's hope the hunters can see well enough to tell the difference between a Canadian soldier and a woodland creature.

To add to the risks we face, the military police informed us that the already high rate of fatal traffic accidents historically triples during the months of October through February. This is a significant issue for our contingent as our soldiers are constantly moving and have driven more than nine hundred thousand kilometres since we have been here – that is a lot of time on the roads.

The personnel handling the weapons count for the various factions panicked the other day because they could not account for fourteen surface-to-air missiles that went missing from one cantonment site. The concern is that these missiles could be headed to Kosovo. Absurdly, when a recount was completed, in addition to finding the fourteen missing missiles, they discovered hundreds of others they didn't even know existed. It sure makes me feel safe knowing that we still have no clue how many deadly weapons the warring factions really have.

4 October 1998

It is the end of week twelve, and the pace of life hasn't slowed down for anyone in senior leadership positions. Today, the monthly Contingent Commander's conference was scheduled at the same time as church services. This is very disappointing as I was very much looking forward to attending another service with our visiting priest. As it turns out, because of the conference and the trip to Medjugorje, only two people attended his service. It must be discouraging to see how little consideration is given to spiritual life here in theatre.

During the conference we were informed that, due to the fighting in Kosovo, some three hundred thousand citizens are living as refugees, with the winter months fast approaching. The Yugoslav army is doing everything in its power to crush the Kosovo Liberation Army, and this includes committing atrocities against innocent women and children. The American and British governments have told their citizens in Yugoslavia and Kosovo to leave ASAP. NATO has moved in all the war assets necessary to perform massive air strikes against Yugoslavia, whose leader simply refuses to comply with the world's demand to stop the fighting. It certainly looks like NATO will begin its air offensive in the next two weeks, at which point who knows what will happen. NATO will likely want to start a land-based offensive shortly after, and we will probably have to provide soldiers and equipment. Our security posture will almost certainly change, as we will become the potential targets of retaliation. The risk of retaliation is difficult to quantify, but it will almost certainly depend on how many Yugoslav citizens are killed in the NATO attacks and on the Yugoslav government's ability to control extremist groups. The biggest question on everyone's mind is why NATO is waiting so long to act in this situation. The damage has already been done, and who else will be able to help the enormous number of refugees who will be forced to endure the harsh winter without food or shelter? Dear Lord, when will we ever learn to stop this kind of senseless killing?

I can imagine my much-anticipated leave being cancelled because I will be needed here. This will be hard to take, especially since my parents are making a special trip to come and see my family and me. The Battle Group played an exhibition soccer game against the British Division HQ this afternoon and won 3–1. It was a great game, and once again I got to enjoy it from the bench. It is experiences like this that serve to remind me that I am not an RCR and will never be included in their close-knit little family. That's OK with me because I already belong to a great family. Good night my loved ones.

---

5 October 1998

This day has just flown by principally because I haven't stopped moving since the time I woke at 0600hrs. If this keeps up, I will be completely exhausted by the time I head home for some much-needed leave. This evening, I found out that the Battle Group's Oscar Company (O Company) paid a visit to the Bihac psychiatric facility, and they will be taking it on as a project. It is truly a worthwhile undertaking, and I am very proud to have been able to facilitate the partnership that will see this work get done. Thank you, Lord, for allowing this to happen. The soldiers of O Company have a great deal to do, but once they are done, they will never forget the contributions they made. I hope these kinds of gestures help to cement in the minds of the Bosnian people that there are a lot of good people out there, and Canadian soldiers are some of the very best. There are enough problems in this country that Canadians could continue to make significant contributions for many years to come.

I was in the clinic all day today and had the chance to see ten patients, which is pretty good for around here. I am starting to get requests for consultations from the other medical officers, and I do enjoy trying to help them diagnose and treat their patients' problems.

I sometimes find myself wishing that I could just be one of the junior medical officers and have the hands-on treatment of patients as my primary duty. Unfortunately, this would be a waste of all the years of experience I have, and it's old goats like me that allow the junior medical officers to dedicate their time to the day-to-day care of our soldiers. I guess we all have our roles to play, and mine is a little more removed from the type of medicine that I enjoy practising.

The Surgeon General's visit continues to be a major time-suck, and I am certain that over the next ten days, it will consume nearly all the time I have and then some. I would like to ensure that he gets a good look at the entire AOR and gets to see Canadian soldiers doing their jobs. We currently have trips planned in an armoured Bison ambulance, a helicopter and a Cougar, and on foot patrols with an infantry company. I just got an e-mail from the big fella himself, and he seems to be quite excited about coming into theatre. I have never been great at hosting people or social events, so I can only hope that he isn't disappointed with what I have put together for him. Only sixteen days till I depart for home, and I can hardly wait to see and hug everyone. Good night my beloved ones.

---

6 October 1998

I had a great day of getting things done today because for some unknown reason, everything I touched didn't turn into crap. I started the day off with a great run in the hills. As I walked to the front gate with the Company Sergeant Major (CSM), he let go a fart that was so powerful, it may have registered on the Richter scale. I couldn't help laughing because I knew half the troops must have heard it, jumped out of their bed and snapped to attention. Little things like this only go to show that even CSMs are human. While we are on the subject of flatus, you will never guess what is on the dinner menu the night before I take my first long road trip with the Surgeon General. If you guessed chili, you win a lifetime supply of methane. Can you imagine the nightmare we'll experience tomorrow morning if I so much as look at a bowl of chili? If my career isn't already on life support, it will be if the Surgeon General dies of respiratory failure in the back of our vehicle. I will definitely have to eat something else on the menu or not eat at all.

We are now down to a core group of approximately eight runners who faithfully get up in the dark and head out to train. I tease the army guys that with the gradual loss of enthusiasm for training, I can feel the growing weakness oozing out of the barracks. This certainly does create a visual image for me.

The intelligence people reported that yesterday some Canadian soldiers who were out for a run were harassed by civilians in a passing car. They were subjected to verbal assaults, and the people in the vehicle rolled down the window and pointed a pistol at them. This is the kind of stuff that scares you, especially when you realize how little respect these folks showed for other ethnic groups during the war years. I am sure that killing a Canadian soldier wouldn't cause them a moment of moral distress.

Today, I drained a seroma (a pocket of fluid) off the leg of a rather shapely young female. It was truly pathetic how the male medical assistants tripped over themselves trying to be helpful. I, of course, maintained an entirely professional demeanour while I spent at least thirty minutes cleaning the site of the seroma prior to doing the aspiration – one can never be too careful about preventing possible infections. Men truly are dogs.

This morning, I noticed for the first time that the abbreviation for my position as medical advisor is MAD, and it's entirely possible I may be completely mad before this tour is over. Many could argue quite convincingly that I didn't have far to go in this respect prior to this deployment.

Fifteen days until I head home to see Janet, the kids, my parents, and the cats, but then who's counting?

---

7 October 1998

One more day until Corporal (Cpl) Stratton and I leave to pick up the grand fromage – the Surgeon General. We have done a great deal of work to coordinate his itinerary. I don't believe this would have been the case if he had been an infantry general officer – in fact, I am certain of it. We will be travelling in a Jeep Cherokee, and I do believe that Cpl Stratton will feel like he has died and gone to driver's heaven. We will be on the road for a whole lot of miles and doing the drive in comfort will certainly help.

One of the Canadians that we will be meeting on our journey asked if we could bring him a twenty-four pack of assorted Canadian beers so that he could give them away as gifts. I suspected this request would not be as easy to grant as it sounded. With the contingent's strict drinking policy, we had to go right to the top for approval, and even then, it was quite awkward. I had somewhat less trouble getting my hands on the seventy-five fire extinguisher tags that he also wanted.

This evening the cooks hosted a medieval supper for the entire camp. The idea was to eat whole chickens, ribs, buns and potatoes with bare hands. While the medical staff found this a novel experience, the infantry lads couldn't figure out what the big deal was because they eat this way all the time. Ouch! Our surgeon came dressed in a wig and skirt and was a big hit with all the lads. For my part, I went to the workshop and crafted a crude sword and brought it along as my butter knife. On the way to the Mess the soldiers were giving both my sword and me strange looks – I assumed it was because of the sword but I may have been mistaken. As I went by them, I told them that the Canadian Armed Forces have run out of money to buy rifles, so they issued me this sword. The scary part of this fabrication is that if the poop ever did hit the fan, I probably would be more effective with a homemade wooden sword than I would with a pistol, based on my pitiful shooting demonstration earlier in the month.

Our surgeon and anaesthetist are almost done their deployments and will be leaving for home in several days. They both appear to be very excited about getting back to their families. I will personally miss them both very much. We have had a lot of fun together and have shared some painful situations during our time here. At the very least I now have two new friends that I might never have made if not for this deployment. In many ways, I wish I were leaving with them. I hope that their replacements are the same calibre of people.

---

8 October 1998

This morning when we left to pick up the Surgeon General, the fog was so thick that you could hardly see your hand in front of your face. Despite the weather, we arrived on time, and what was even more impressive was that I was navigating, and we didn't get lost for even the briefest of moments. General Auger and Chief Warrant Officer (CWO) Doucet both looked somewhat tired from their twelve-hour journey, but our schedule demanded that they visit a few places before they could rack out.

Things started off with a visit to Zagreb's trauma hospital where, unfortunately, the recent war has provided the staff with ample opportunity to develop considerable expertise in acute trauma management. During the war, they apparently treated over two thousand major trauma cases and over ten thousand less significant injuries. The staff have an obvious passion for their work, but their facility falls well below the standard one would expect for similar institutions in North America.

From there we went to the Forensic Science Centre where we met one of the forensic medicine specialists who are doing a great deal of work to identify human remains being exhumed from mass gravesites. This is painstaking work, and in many cases, they must resort to DNA analysis to establish a victim's identity. They can use techniques whereby they extract DNA from bone and teeth. Very few laboratories in the world have this capability. The professor showed us examples of tattooed skin that had survived for nearly seven years in a mass gravesite. He also showed us pictures of the charred remains of older persons who had been tied to a chair and lit on fire. The remains of the individuals were virtually welded to the parts of the chair that survived the blaze. It's hard to imagine that people could be so cruel to each other.

We ended the day by going out to a nice restaurant and eating a traditional Croatian meal. General Auger asked a lot of questions about a wide variety of topics and certainly appears to be sincerely interested in learning more about what serving in this theatre of operations is all about. I have taken the hospital's digital camera with me and am really enjoying taking photographs of everything we see. It will be interesting to be able to share these with the folks back home. Day one of the visit down and only six more to survive. Hooah!

---

9 October 1998

It is Friday in theatre and what that means is there are only two more working days until Monday. The first meeting scheduled for this morning was with Dr. Gluhinic, the Croatian Assistant Minister of Health. Dr. Gluhinic is a chain-smoking former orthopaedic surgeon who seemed to have his own agenda for our meeting. We were surprised to discover that there were formal agreements between SFOR and the Government of Croatia that reference the provision of health care to SFOR soldiers. On the other hand, he was surprised to discover that for several years now we have had a Croatian medical liaison (Dr. Igor Begovic) whom he had never met or even heard of. He did not seem overly pleased to hear this – I hope Igor does not get into trouble as a result.

This morning while doing my ablutions, I decided to trim my moustache with the trimmer I had received last Christmas. Unfortunately, I forgot to put on the guide and nearly cut off the entire right side of my moustache. The only way around it was to cut the rest of my moustache the same length and hope the general didn't notice my facial transformation. To my disappointment, one of the first things he noted was the wretched state of my much diminished moustache, but when I told him my story, we all had a good laugh.

I discovered today that the Canadian REMFs who are stationed in Croatia refer to the operational theatre in Bosnia as "the Box." They are quick to point out that, while they live a Holiday Inn lifestyle outside of the Box, they do not get paid as much as those of us who work inside the Box. Gee, that sure makes me feel a lot better about the whole thing. I am glad I don't work there because they are not getting the operational experience that I am.

The contingent has just been ordered to increase its alert status to Black Tango Charlie in anticipation of problems related to Kosovo. In this alert state we are not allowed to exercise outside the camp unless we are wearing our flak jacket and load-bearing vest and are carrying a loaded weapon. Wouldn't that make for a fun run? I sure hope this doesn't last for too long or I will get very sick of running around in tiny circles within the dusty confines of Stalag Coralici. It is likely that NATO will issue an activation order tomorrow and then who knows what will happen.

We escorted the Surgeon General into the Box this afternoon and were expected back for a guard of honour for the general at 1530hrs.

We arrived at precisely 1530hrs, so the troops were not forced to stand for too long awaiting our arrival. I do not believe that General Auger is used to all this attention, and I think at times he would rather be just one of the boys. Everyone thinks that the digital camera is great, and by some miracle I managed to successfully download all of today's shots onto the computer. If this continues, I will leave the theatre a techno-weenie and not simply a weenie.

Janet is attending a sport medicine conference today, and I cannot help but be jealous of her. I hope she brings home some good free swag.

10 October 1998

Day three of the Surgeon General's visit, and all appears to be going well. We started the day off with a tour of the National Support Element – essentially the folks that support the sharp enders so they can effectively do their jobs. The big fella was then taken by Bison ambulance up to the ambulanta (clinic) in Todorovo. The weather was great, and he had the opportunity to see some of the inspiring geography that is so typical of this area of Bosnia. Once again, Cpl Stratton absolutely nailed the timing for the quarter guard that awaited General Auger when he arrived in Stalag Coralici.

In Coralici, General Auger was accorded great hospitality, which essentially translated to him having to endure a wide variety of briefings. Unfortunately for him, having been in theatre only a few days, he hardly understood a word the presenters said – I know the feeling all too well. O Company took us out on a foot patrol through the town of Cazin, and that gave me the opportunity to ride in another armoured vehicle. Since we were travelling in a convoy consisting of a Bison and a Grizzly, I had a choice. Despite everyone recommending I ride in the Bison because it is the better vehicle,

I elected to try the Grizzly since I had never been in one before. The Grizzly is a twenty-foot-long, six-wheeled, ten-ton, armoured personnel carrier. I ended up with the last laugh as the Bison broke down shortly after we left the camp, and everyone had to be crammed into the Grizzly.

The day ended with a tour of the medical facilities and a party in the ASC stand-easy tent. In a well-intentioned and innocent attempt to invite her fellow officers to attend this event, the CO of the ASC announced at the mess, "You are all invited over to the ASC tonight where we will show you a real good time in our tent." It took the CO and the entire officers mess all of about a microsecond to realize what she had said, and it took another microsecond for her to turn red as a beet. I am afraid she will be hearing about this well-intended announcement for a very long time.

In addition to my role as the Surgeon General's aide-de-camp, I am also functioning as a photo documentarian extraordinaire. It is not uncommon for romantic relations to develop when people work for prolonged periods in intense environments, and I am ashamed to admit that I have succumbed to "temptations of the flash." For whatever reason, I am falling head over heels in love with the digital camera I am allowed to use. I especially like being able to download the photos I have taken onto the computer's hard drive and then simply carry on.

I have been falling asleep in the car while dragging the Surgeon General from place to place. Yesterday, everyone in the car was having a great laugh because I kept bashing my head into the window and didn't appear to notice. I reassured them that it is difficult to hurt something that is largely empty and seldom ever used. If my head is truly that empty, then I may have the potential for further advancement in the military.

11 October 1998

Day four of the Surgeon General's visit is over, and everything continues to go tickety-boo. Our initial visit was to the Para Company platoon house just outside the town of Bosanski Petrovac. The soldiers love living there, but for the life of me, I can't understand why. Not only does the place lack running water, outdoor showers and heat, but also only 25 percent of it has any form of roof over top of it. The soldiers living there describe the place as a Bob Vila special. In my opinion, it looks more like a demolition special. I guess for soldiers used to living in the field, this dilapidated old shack is a little piece of heaven. By comparison, the luxurious accommodations at Stalag Coralici are looking better and better.

Following this, we travelled to Drvar where the boss got to meet the medical staff. He was then given an account – the abbreviated VIP version – of the riots which rocked this town in April '98. Man, did the citizens ever go on a rampage. They destroyed the police station and burned the police cars and fire trucks. They then went through a large apartment complex beating up and evicting 120 Serbian families who were living there. Finally, they confronted a company of Canadian soldiers, and as a result, several of our soldiers were injured by the rocks and bottles thrown at them. Ultimately, the Company Commander felt his troops were under so much threat that he fired his pistol over the head of the rioters. If anything, this only made things worse, and it wasn't until one of the soldiers fired off a machine gun that people finally decided to back off. Thank goodness no one was shot during this altercation because this would almost certainly have created years of problems for SFOR troops.

The last place we went to see was the camp in Zgon. After several more briefings, we had the opportunity to tour the unit medical station, and I was very impressed by the professional layout that they have. In the evening, we went on a foot patrol through the town of Kljuc. The day concluded with a beer in the Mess and an opportunity to spend several hours discussing what the medical staff see as trade-related issues. What impressed me the most today was the can-do attitude of our troops and the ingenuity of our engineers. The platoon house operates out of a blown-up storage building, Camp Drvar is set up in a decommissioned bakery and some grain silos, and our camp in Zgon is housed in an old carpet factory. Despite lacking many of the basic services that we take for granted back in Canada, the average soldier seems very happy to be helping to bring peace to this region. I am taking lots of pictures to show others what these places look like so that they can have a better idea of what the hell I am talking about.

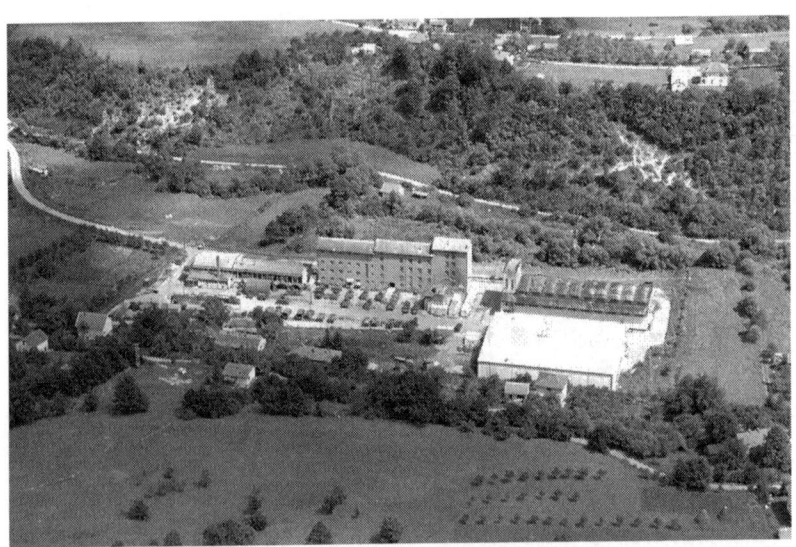

Camp Drvar, affectionately referred to as Castle Grey Skull by the soldiers who lived there.

12 October 1998

We had a very busy day of travelling and visiting today, and everyone is looking a bit worn out. Our itinerary included tours of the surgical facilities in Sipovo (British), Novi Travnik (Dutch) and Rajlovac (German). At each location, the Surgeon General was given a comprehensive look at what our medical colleagues have to offer and the opportunity to ask a lot of pointed questions. We spent a lot of time on the road driving from one place to the next, and the boss accused me of using the long rides as a rather blatant attempt to get him to quit smoking.

The pistol I have to carry with me comes with a holster and leg strap. I find the leg strap constricting when I sit for too long, and so I regularly undo it. When I got up from our briefing in Sipovo I stood up and reached into my groin to locate my leg strap. Unbeknownst to me, the female British anaesthetist was watching all of this and asked, "Whatever are you doing?" When I responded that I was simply trying to locate my accoutrements she smiled and said, "So that's what you call them in Canada."

I have been falling asleep for a fifteen-minute power nap at approximately 1430hrs every day. As my travelling compadres have informed me, when this happens my head bobs all over the place and I regularly bang into the window of our vehicle. The Surgeon General figures that by the time his visit is over, I should be entitled to a medical pension for repetitive cervical spine trauma. He may be right.

In Sarajevo, we were graciously hosted by LCol Van Hootegem – a Dutch officer working with the Medical Coordination Centre. None of us can pronounce his name, so I have started calling him "LCol Hooters" and the nickname seems to have stuck. This evening, he took us into downtown Sarajevo to see the massive amount of damage that was done during the war as well as the infamous Sniper

Alley. Unfortunately for many, this was a main thoroughfare and had to be travelled on to do simple things like shopping or going to work. We went downtown in LCol Hooter's compact car and had to fit CWO Doucet, Cpl Stratton and me into a space in which two normal-sized people would feel uncomfortable. Cpl Stratton is a huge man, and when he finally managed to squeeze himself into the car, he ended up sitting on my pistol. I apologized for giving him a 9mm enema and he indicated that this was great news because his initial concern was that I was happy to see him.

One of the things we have noticed about the people of Bosnia is that they wear a great deal of black clothing, and I suspect this is likely because most of it is purchased on the "black" market.

The General was housed for the night in Camp Ilidza, which is the SFOR headquarters although it looks more like a Holiday Inn resort than a military camp. The rest of us slugs had to sleep in Camp Butmir. We were all given rooms to share with three complete strangers and no bedsheets, blankets or pillows. We chose instead to sleep in our Works and Design section's TV room where once again I was given the opportunity for some much-needed beauty sleep on a well-worn couch.

----

13 October 1998

The morning began with a meeting with the theatre surgeon, Colonel Doctor Wolfgang Weinhart. He spent two hours explaining to us what he and his largely unnecessary staff did for SFOR. We were also introduced to a French major general and a logistics colonel who also do very little to help the troops who work at the sharp end do their job better. One of the major objectives of the SFOR headquarters is to look at ways to reduce the size of the NATO force deployed in Bosnia without reducing its operational effectiveness. When we left there, the Surgeon

General and I both agreed that the first big savings could be achieved by eliminating the entire headquarters staff. The only reason anyone might know they were gone would be the decrease in alcohol consumed and the increase in real work accomplished.

It took us five hours to drive from Sarajevo to Banja Luka to see the Divisional Surgeon and his staff. The scenery on the mountainous roadways was breathtakingly beautiful. We drove through mountain tunnel after mountain tunnel, and the narrow roads and daredevil Bosnian drivers made for numerous close calls. When we finally arrived in Banja Luka, two Challenger main battle tanks were guarding the front gate, while a group of soldiers were busy building sandbag barriers. We suspected that something was up and found out that NATO had signed the activation orders for an attack on the Serbs, and in response, our division has decided to further elevate our alert state. We are now required to travel in convoys of two vehicles or more, everyone in the vehicles must be armed, and each vehicle must have at least one rifle. We can no longer leave the base to go for a run at all, and the black-market CD shops are out of bounds. As an extra measure, the external lighting in the camp is being turned off at night to provide a lower optical signature. This doesn't make a great deal of sense to me as the camp has been here for years, and all the bad guys know exactly where it is located. What the blackout does do is create a situation whereby it is very hazardous to even walk around – I am surprised no one has ended up breaking a leg yet.

Banja Luka is a predominantly British unit whose personnel certainly have a very active mess life. There was a crowd of some forty people or more in the mess before supper, and they remained there until well past 2300hrs. Their drinking rule is entirely open, with the exception that if you drink too much and are unable to function the next day, they will hang you. British standards for the treatment of their personnel still reflect archaic British class system values compared to Canadian standards. Their officers get fed substantially better than their NCMs (non-commissioned members), and their quarters are also of much higher quality. I was so distressed about where our NCM driver, Cpl Stratton, was going to be housed, that I had him sleep in my room where he would at least have some warmth and quiet.

The highlight of my day was watching a young Canadian captain play poke chest with the Surgeon General over the issue of teaching soldiers to be able to administer IVs. The captain felt that the soldiers could practice on each other every week and that this would also help to make them tougher. It took a great deal of restraint for me not to tell him that I thought he was a complete idiot.

----

14 October 1998

Regrettably, the remainder of the Surgeon General's visit has been hijacked by the situation developing in Kosovo. As a result, we headed back to Coralici today in a convoy of three vehicles. During the journey, we encountered a crowd blocking the road we were travelling on. Without saying anything, Cpl Stratton and I simultaneously placed a clip into our weapons, locked all the doors and rolled up all the windows. Unbeknownst to us, these people were shopping at a large roadside marketplace and harboured no ill intent. We enjoyed a nice lunch in Coralici, and the boss got to say his final goodbyes to the surgical staff.

We had to drive up to VK in a convoy so that the general could complete his clearances and debrief the Contingent Commander. We headed for Zagreb at 1500hrs and made it into town just in time for rush hour traffic – oh what a joy. Zagreb is huge but poorly laid out, with very few street signs. Despite this, we only got lost once. That is about as good as it gets when I am the navigator. Cpl Stratton has driven nearly two thousand kilometres over very demanding terrain in the last seven days, and he looked very tired this evening. We had a nice dinner at a local Italian restaurant and called it quits early so that we could all have some time to recharge.

I was very pleased with how the Surgeon General's visit went. Apparently, the Surgeon General saw everything important in theatre and still managed to enjoy himself. I hope General Auger returns home from Bosnia with a greater understanding of the dynamics of this theatre of operations and employs this information to better help the medical team play their supporting role. This trip provided me with the unique opportunity to ask the leader of the Canadian Forces medical world a wide variety of questions, and I do believe that our people are in very capable hands.

---

15 October 1998

The weather has been absolutely awesome for the last while, which sure made it easier to host the Surgeon General. This morning, we delivered the big boss safely to the airport for his long journey back to Canada. It will be my turn to make the same journey in a week, and I am really in need of some hugs and kisses from my loved ones. Accompanying the Surgeon General during his visit helped me to realize just how much I have learned in the four months that I have been here. When we said goodbye, he looked me in the eye and said, "It is unfortunate that we never deployed you into an operational theatre years ago, as your career would likely have gone a long way." I chose not to mention that I have never been asked to deploy before and that, although I have been asking – for six years – to learn to speak French, this doesn't seem to be achievable. It is unfortunate that our "so called" career management system often fails to enhance the capabilities of many of our best assets.

I have returned from this visit feeling somewhat changed, and the staff have been telling me, "We missed you, Dad." I also missed them

– it is nice to be part of a team that is working well to take care of patients. The hectic schedule has left Cpl Stratton and me exhausted and in need of a few stable days living in Stalag Coralici. We decided to take a relaxed trip home and ended up encountering a series of road construction projects that delayed our arrival by forty-five minutes. We must have been extremely tired because the construction delays didn't appear to bother either of us. Ordinarily we both would have sat in our seats and fumed.

The Kosovo situation seems to have settled down somewhat with that murdering SOB Milosevic finally giving in to pressure from NATO. The tragic part is that he only gave in after his troops committed the same atrocities that ravaged this part of the world not that many years ago. We are all hoping that this peace will last because SFOR's job will be infinitely more difficult should it not. The local violence continues, however, with a homemade bomb being used to blow up a vehicle in one of the towns we monitor.

Someone recently told me a joke that exemplifies the situation in Bosnia. A farmer who had lost most of what he owned during the war was out walking his field when he struck something metal with his foot. Fearing it was a land mine, he bent over only to discover it was the kind of lamp that genies come out of in storybooks. Feeling somewhat foolish, he gave it a few rubs, and to his amazement a genie appeared and offered him the classic three wishes. The farmer thought about all his days of hunger and used his first wish to request a huge banquet of his favourite foods and beverages, which the genie granted. For his second wish, the farmer asked for a beautiful new automobile, and the genie produced a 1998 BMW sedan in his favourite colour. After carefully considering his last wish, the farmer stated that, while he dearly loved his wife, to be truthful she wasn't very attractive. He asked the genie if he could make her beautiful. The genie said this might be possible, but he would need to see a picture of her first. When the genie saw the picture of her, he jumped back in shock, never having seen a woman who was quite so gruesome looking. The genie explained to the farmer that making his wife more attractive would be extremely difficult, and it would be better to make another wish. The farmer was very disappointed and said the only other thing he would like to see was peace in Bosnia. When the genie heard this, he quickly asked if he could see the picture of the man's wife once more.

---

16 October 1998

Only six more sleeps until I get to go home and see my loved ones. I sure hope they haven't forgotten what I look like. It's funny to see the different emotions that people experience when they come back from being on leave. Surprisingly, many of them are very happy because they feel strangely lost while they are away, even if the time is spent with their families. Others find it very hard to come back knowing it's going to be months before they will see their families again. For these folks it's almost like they are going away twice instead of having a little break during one lengthy period of absence. It is amazing how differently we all react to the pressures in our lives.

Today, I spent my time trying to straighten up all the crap that accumulated while I was away with the big boss guy. While I tried really hard, at the end of the day it doesn't appear that I have much to show for all my efforts. Perhaps I will do better tomorrow.

I have been taking pictures since coming here, and I now have over five hundred digital images saved in a zip file. This will allow me to share this experience with others, which I think is a very important thing to do. Our public affairs officer returned from having spent her three weeks' leave with her husband in Greece. She looked bronzed and well rested. While she was away, her photographer broke his left wrist. When she walked into her office, her mischievous co-workers informed her that I had decided that her photographer was unfit to remain in theatre and would have to be replaced. They even conducted a brief medal presentation for him. To add icing to the cake, his replacement was supposed to be some "nightmare" photo tech. They let poor Captain Chaloux stew over this for several hours before they finally told her that it was all a big joke and that her photographer would be staying. She was so happy she forgot all about how awful it was coming back to work in Bosnia after frying on the beaches of Greece for twenty-one days. I had the photographer digitally manipulate a photograph for me that I hope to surprise the Battle Group Commander with at tomorrow's big team briefing. I sure hope he still has his sense of humour, or my next posting will likely be somewhere not so warm – like the North Pole. Stay tuned.

---

17 October 1998

I am starting to let myself get excited about going home, but I must try to remember that I still have a job to do here. It will be so nice to see everyone again and tell them that I missed them.

Many soldiers are now starting to come and see me with their orthopaedic injuries or for training advice. This is very encouraging as it suggests to me that they are finally beginning to accept me as part of the team. Either that or they are so desperate that they are willing to take their chances on an old fart like me. As part of my indoctrination into the group, I am continuing to try to improve my ability to speak a second language – Armyese. Armyese is a unique dialect that consists of a combination of acronyms and cuss words. What I am concerned about is returning home and having no one understand what I am saying – not that this really matters because no one there listens to anything I say anyway.

This morning, I had the intelligence section help me load my secret picture into a PowerPoint presentation that I could use at the weekly Battle Group briefing. The picture was taken during the Surgeon General's visit when we coaxed the Contingent Commander and the CO of the Battle Group to put on these goofy-looking surgical hats and pretend that they were performing surgery on our anaesthetist. The picture turned out magnificently. Much to the chagrin of the Battle Group's CO, I told him that wearing a surgical hat, he bears a close resemblance to Yasser Arafat. You can imagine how much he loved to hear that. Yesterday, when the photo tech and I were playing around with this particular photo, I suddenly realized that the Contingent Commander was holding the gas mask on our fake patient and the CO of the Battle Group was pretending to be the surgeon. Given this convenient arrangement I decided to title the photo "The Gasser and Yasser."

The CO's briefing this afternoon was rather routine. The only amusing part was when the lawyer and padre indicated that they would be teaching their replacements how to behave properly during these briefings, to prevent any embarrassing moments in the future. During these briefings, everyone in the room is given the opportunity to raise any points they feel the group should know about, and today I happened to be the second last person to speak. After mentioning a few minor issues, I concluded by informing everyone that we had just had a rotation of our surgical team (which was true) and that I thought I would use a photograph to introduce the new surgical team since, as we all know, a picture paints a thousand words. When I put the slide up on the screen, the entire room burst into uproarious laughter that lasted for quite some time. When everyone settled down, I told the CO that, with his permission, I would be all too happy to instruct the replacement padre and lawyer on how to properly behave during briefings. I sense that he will not likely take me up on this generous offer. The CO took it very well, and I suspect he will be seeking vengeance in the near future. On his way out of the mess this evening, he mentioned to me that he would be suggesting to the Contingent Commander the need for physician services on our remote radio re-broadcasting station on top of

Mount Gola and that I would be an ideal candidate for the job. Moments later he returned with a huge grin on his face and reminded me that, since Col Natynczyk was away for the next three weeks, he was in fact the Contingent Commander. I have always wanted to see Mount Gola, and now it looks like I may even get a chance to live there. Hooah! It is wonderful to work with leaders who can take a well-intended joke and respond with a few shots of their own.

18 October 1998

While I had great plans for the day, I did not get nearly as much done as I set out to accomplish. Things began to unravel at about 0900hrs when the United Nations International Police Task Force brought us one of their officers who had just had a seizure in his car. This was the first time the fellow had ever experienced such a problem, and I think it may have had something to do with the fact that he had worked forty-seven days in a row, only had three-and-a-half-hours' sleep the night before and did not have any breakfast. We admitted him and will be heli-evacing him to the German field hospital in Sarajevo tomorrow morning.

When we call the German field hospital, it is truly impressive to hear how many of their staff speak English, although some communication errors do occur. For instance, this morning I asked to speak to the neurologist. When the doctor came to the phone, I outlined the entire case for him, indicating that I felt the police officer needed a consultation, an EEG (electroencephalogram) and a CT scan. When I had finished, he told me that he was a urologist and questioned why I wasn't sending the patient to a neurologist. While this mix-up in communication was purely accidental, it may in fact have been quite appropriate given that some males seem to have their brains located in their pants.

Last night, I received an awesome care package from my parents. It contained most of the essentials for survival: jujubes, power bars, and not just ordinary jellybeans but Jelly Belly beans, the Cadillac of jellybeans. The package also contained a beautiful crucifix that is now hanging in our humble chapel and greatly appreciated by everyone in our tiny congregation.

Last night we were instructed to move our clocks back one hour as part of the annual daylight savings strategy. Everyone thought this was somewhat unusual because this time change doesn't occur in Canada until next week. Tonight we were told to put our clocks one hour forward as somebody screwed up and got the dates for the change wrong. I am so confused now I am no longer sure what day let alone what hour it is.

Two ladies from the ASC staff were out enjoying a fitness walk late this afternoon when someone in a vehicle flashed an AK-47 in their direction. They reported the incident and then spent the evening patrolling around with the Battle Group in a futile attempt to identify the vehicle. This is the same type of intimidation that is being used on the local people. I wonder how long such stupidity will continue.

As I mentioned before, military personnel who are not employed in Bosnia frequently refer to Bosnia as the Box. I suppose that if your first name happens to be Jack and you are deployed to Bosnia, we should technically refer to you as a "Jack in the Box." Triple ouch!

I have just been informed that I will be the most senior Canadian on our return flight to Canada next week and am therefore responsible for the behaviour of all the other Canadian Forces personnel on the aircraft. This is just the kind of babysitting job that I was hoping for, to ensure that the start of my leave will be oh so very special. Four more days and counting.

19 October 1998

It has rained pretty much all day and that sure can put a damper on things – pardon the pun. This morning the British medical evacuation team arrived to pick up the police officer we had admitted to our ASC after his seizure. It is amazing to see all the multinational cooperation that occurs around here. In this particular case, an American police officer was taken to a Canadian medical facility and then transferred by a British helicopter to a German field hospital. Think of what the world would be like if we could do this on a global scale. Maybe we would end up fighting with each other a lot less.

My CD player began misbehaving several days ago, and today it finally stopped working altogether. I am rather disappointed because I really do enjoy listening to a wide variety of tunes while working late at night. My problem is that I don't have a clue where to get it repaired here.

The CO of the Battle Group has been giving me wary looks since I bladed him at his last briefing. Given this gentleman's personality, I fear that it will not be long before he gets even with me in some insidious way. If I do not end up as the medical officer for the six soldiers working in isolation at the top of Mount Gola, it might be something more challenging like an all-expense paid visit to the Crowbar Hotel in Edmonton. Who knows, maybe my parents who happen to live in Edmonton will get to visit me once in a while and bring me extra bread and water.

The harmony of any unit is dependent on the personalities of the people involved. It took awhile, but the previous surgical team finally came together and was a great deal of fun to work with. Our new surgical team is quite different. The surgeon is a recent graduate and is somewhat uncertain about how everything works around here. The anaesthetist is on his fourth tour and is private to the point of appearing to be aloof. In an effort to be welcoming, we invited both of them to come out and play basketball with us. The surgeon declined on the grounds that he cannot afford to injure his hands. The anaesthetist, on the other hand, elected to play and proceeded to foul everyone within striking distance. It wasn't intentional, he simply didn't seem to realize that basketball isn't a collision sport. It will take some time, but I hope our new surgical team becomes as close as the last one.

Yesterday, we were informed that there would be no other opportunities to visit Medjugorje. This change in attitude likely stems from a fear that if the Canadian media ever found out that some of our soldiers were being given a day and a half off to visit a religious shrine, there would be hell to pay with the Canadian public. It doesn't matter that those same soldiers are working twelve to fourteen hours per day, seven days a week, for the same pay they earn back in Canada. It sure makes you wonder! Mother Mary, please keep my loved ones in your prayers. Amen.

---

20 October 1998

It has rained for the second straight day, which has kept us all huddled up inside. I imagine this is what the winter months are going to be like around here.

Captain Liz Davis visited our humble camp this morning. She is an American military physician from the 525th Expeditionary Military Unit located in Zagreb. She is coming to see some of the Box and the medical facilities available in this theatre. In her mind, it makes more sense for the nations in theatre to pool their resources so we can be less dependent on the Croatian medical system, which is becoming less and less welcoming towards SFOR patients. It has been my experience that this is a rather unusual attitude for an American medical person in this theatre, as the American military tends to be very insular. I like her approach – it is one we have been using throughout our deployment. Captain Davis informed me that the Americans have a hospital in Aviano, Italy, that has just about every bell and whistle a medical person could ever want access to. I would like to visit this place to determine if our medical team can start sending some of our people there.

Yesterday a deminer was killed trying to rid this place of one of the millions of land mines that were put into the ground during the war. Tragically, he is one of over fifty people who are killed or badly maimed by land mines every month in Bosnia. Since 1996, over six hundred children in Bosnia have been the victims of mine warfare. It is estimated that there are more than six million land mines scattered around Bosnia in more than eighteen thousand different minefields – unbelievable! With those kinds of numbers, I am afraid that we will continue to see innocent people being badly injured by mines for many years to come. The UN estimates that Bosnia is only the tip of the iceberg and that, worldwide, over one hundred million land mines are lying in wait to hurt innocent people. I think that Lady Di was way ahead of her time in trying to get these senselessly destructive weapons banned from use.

This afternoon, we also had visitors from the Jesuit Refugee Service come to ask if they could use our medical expertise to help them assess children who have been injured by mines to determine their future treatment needs. Our surgeon is very keen to get involved and so am I. I hope that the big cheeses of the world will permit us to get involved in this worthwhile work.

The Army continues to provide me with interesting lessons. Today I learned a new term for a wife. "Niner" is the military designation for a commanding officer, and so the term for an army wife is a "niner domestic." I don't think my niner domestic would tolerate being called a niner domestic for very long.

It is time to head home for a while as I find myself wearing my uniform for longer and longer periods each day. If this keeps up, I will soon be sleeping in my uniform.

21 October 1998

This is the last day I will spend in theatre for a while, and it
started out in grand fashion. Just as the group that I was running
with entered the front gate, the power to the entire camp went out.
This meant two important things to me: no warmth in any room in
the camp and ice-cold shower water. For whatever reason, I did not
get to enjoy an even slightly warm shower any day this week. To
make matters somewhat more complex, we ended up seeing a fair
number of patients today, leaving me very little time to make all
those last-minute preparations that one always needs to make before going on a trip. I normally use an electric shaver, but because
of the power failure, I was forced to use a manual razor. As I was
shaving in the men's washroom with all the virile army types, I realized to my absolute horror that I was using a lady's razor. To their
considerable credit, the guys told me they didn't mind this, as long
as I didn't insist on using it to shave my legs. Several "Grey Men"
have suggested that I consider getting involved in the world of the
"Secret Squirrels" – the joint task force. To be truthful, I think it

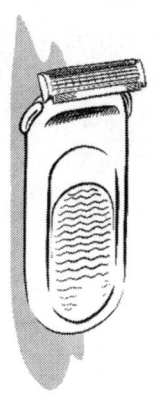

My lady's razor

would be awesome to work with this elite military unit as long as I get to keep my lady's razor.

Captain Edora and I filmed a quick tour of the camp using his video camera. We went everywhere and considering that we were doing this thing off the top of our heads, I think it turned out pretty well. I hope the video will help give my family a better idea of what life here is all about.

This evening, we left Stalag Coralici on what the drivers affectionately refer to as the "happy bus" – every bus taking you home safe and sound is a happy bus. My guess is that the buses bringing people back from leave must be referred to as the "sad buses." As I prepare for my long-anticipated break from Stalag Coralici, I am feeling mixed emotions. On the one hand, I am very excited to be getting home to my family, but on the other hand, I will definitely miss the adopted family that I have been living with here in theatre.

When we arrived in VK this evening, we discovered that the heater was not working in the building where we would be sleeping. Nothing says "enjoy your vacation" like sleeping in a refrigerator. I was also quickly introduced to the corporal responsible for briefing our group about the preparations for our departure and all the rules by which we must abide. He informed me that as the senior military person on the flight, I was required to read a statement outlining my responsibilities to ensure that all the soldiers on our flight behave themselves. I was then introduced to the entire group, and they were all told that I was the one who would be addressing them should they get into trouble. I don't anticipate we will have any problems.

---

22 October 1998

We were up today at 0500hrs to depart on our grand journey home. Everyone was very excited so most of us slept poorly, if it all. This was likely due to a combination of the anticipation of returning to our loved ones and the freezing temperatures in our accommodations. It is amazing how much more uncomfortable sleeping on a concrete floor is when the floor is ice-cold. I slept in one of the medical offices with a medical assistant from Coralici, and even with a space heater we were both chilled to the bone. The trip to Zagreb was uneventful, and I spent most of it sprawled out on the front seat. Our itinerary shows that the trip will take twenty-four hours and includes stops in Frankfurt and Toronto. I can't express how much I love wasting time in airports.

When we were landing in Frankfurt, I noticed that the airfield was surrounded by a beautiful forest, and knowing the German people, this forest would almost certainly be criss-crossed with groomed fitness trails. The temptation to sneak in a running workout on German soil was overwhelming, and so I toddled off down the road in search of a way out of the airport's concrete jungle and into the trees. To my amazement, I only had to walk about ten minutes and hop a large fence to achieve my goal. I then had to find some dense bush so that I could change into my running stuff and hide my clothing and carry-on luggage. I managed this without being arrested for exposing myself in public and was rewarded with a wonderful workout on some amazing fitness trails. Just as I was finishing my run, it began to rain, and so I had a shower au naturel to boot. When I finally returned to the airport, I was happy to find that no one had taken my stuff, as it would have been an unpleasant flight home in a soaking wet T-shirt and shorts. Who says I'm an exercise addict?

When we arrived in Toronto, half of us discovered we had not been checked through to Ottawa and the flights to Ottawa were over-booked. After some tense moments, all but one soldier made it on the plane, and I am certain he made it onto the 2200hrs flight.

Janet was at the airport to meet me, and it sure was nice to be able to hug my wife for the first time in months. It will take me awhile to get used to walking on grass, not seeing weapons everywhere and not looking out at the world through barbed wire fences. Thank you, Lord, for getting us all home safely!

Leave Summary

As my leave period rapidly draws to a close, I now have the opportunity to reflect on how it actually went. While twenty-one days sounds like a long time, it seemed to pass in the blink of an eye. It was great to get home and touch base with reality even if it was all too briefly. While this break is called leave, for many of us it turns out to be an opportunity to jam as much life into a three-week period as humanly possible. I have always lived life this way and this visit was no exception.

I had a chance to watch Janet's convocation after six very hard years of university training. She graduated cum laude with a bachelor's degree in science and a special certificate of competency as a nurse practitioner. This is quite an accomplishment for a mother of three who works in emergency medicine and helps to coordinate the smooth functioning of our sport medicine clinic. The graduation ceremony was very moving, and I must admit that I felt exceptionally privileged to share this important day with my special lady.

We also had the chance to enjoy a week with my parents, who flew in on the 28th of October. My parents are very special people, and given the health problems that my mother has recently endured, it was wonderful to see her looking so well. She is walking on her own and is still as sharp as a tack. Dad also looks very well and has matured into a superb cook.

In a moment of insanity, Dad and I headed off to the Dwyer Hill Training Centre to visit "Those of Whom We Dare Not Speak." Unfortunately for us, on the day we went, the *Ottawa Citizen* published a front-page article outlining the activities of Canada's secret soldiers. When we arrived at the gate, the security stance was quite high, and while they would allow me in with an escort, they would not allow my father to enter the base. I told Dad that he was denied because of his "beady little eyes," but the truth was that the senior staff were very upset about this article and were being far more restrictive than usual about who gets a chance to tour this highly secretive unit. I really could not blame them, but I was very disappointed because I know that my father would truly have enjoyed the experience.

Dr. Chris Georgantopoulus has been working very hard to maintain my medical practice in my absence, and he really needed a break while I was home. During my three weeks' leave, I ended up seeing patients at seven evening clinics, and it was nice to get back into the swing of things. It was also very nice to see many of my patients and friends. They seem to like "Dr. G" a great deal, and maybe when I return, we can continue to share the practice. This might allow us both to enjoy clinical medicine without being worked to death.

What seemed to dominate a great deal of my precious time at home was humanitarian aid for Bosnia. Things started out simply enough, but as the days went on, they seemed to snowball to the point that we were having trouble keeping up with the demands. The cause is very worthwhile but unfortunately, it cut deeply into the private time that I would have liked to enjoy with my family. Janet is a woman of considerable patience, but I know I left her at the airport disappointed that we did not have more private moments together. I am not sure what we could have done differently, but I hope she knows how truly special she is to me.

When all was said and done, I ended up giving five public presentations and four media interviews and did a whole lot of running around. The community raised $4,144.97 and donated approximately sixty boxes of winter clothing. Ontario Medical Supply let us buy our medical supplies at cost and then donated an additional $15,000 worth of medical items. A family friend, Ginette Jarvo, and I delivered two Dodge Caravans full of supplies to the 3 RCR BG building in Petawawa. I ended up getting on the plane in Ottawa not knowing how or if these generous donations would ever make their way to Coralici.

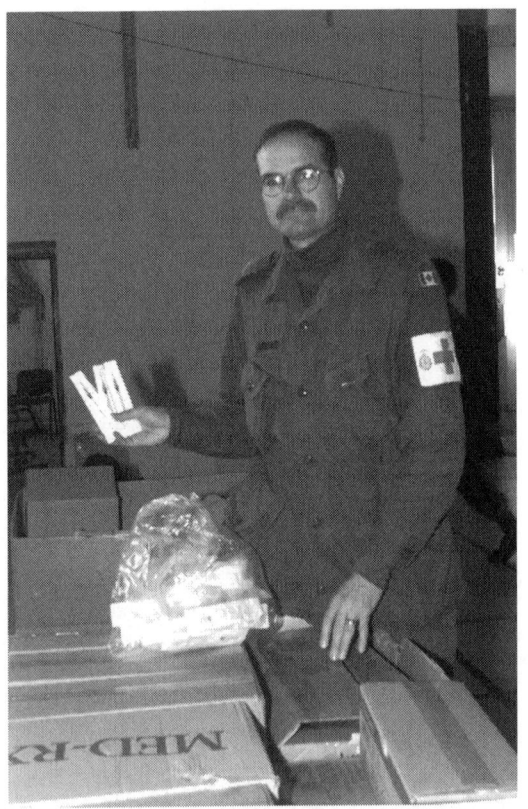

(With permission from Darrell Menard)

Medical supplies that were purchased with donations from the generous people of Russell, Ontario. After considerable effort, these supplies were eventually transported to Bosnia on Canadian Armed Forces aircraft

November 1998

12 November 1998

It is 2300hrs and I have just arrived back in Stalag Coralici. I now fully understand why the drivers refer to the buses that bring them back from leave as the sad buses. Boy, what a sombre crowd we were. There was no laughing, no smiling and very little conversation. The journey was actually rather depressing, and I think this accurately reflected the general mood of our group. I, for one, found it more difficult to say goodbye this time around than I did in July. Janet and I both cried in each other's arms, and I found it very difficult to let go of her. At a moment like this, you sure begin to wonder if all the pain of being apart from the people you love most is really worth it.

During the trip back I had the opportunity to reflect on how my leave went, and I was struck by the amount of activity we managed to jam into twenty-one days. It was disappointing to realize that I did not spend as much time with my wife as she deserved. While raising funds for medical supplies to send to Bosnia was important, it made it challenging to find much special time to spend together. I sure hope that when I return to Canada in February things will be quieter.

The trip back took a total of twenty-two hours and once again involved a five-hour layover in Frankfurt, Germany. I used this opportunity to do a ninety-minute workout in the same beautiful forest adjacent to the airport. This little moment with nature turned out to be the high point of my trip. The Germans sure do make good use of their forests.

For the return trip, I was once again the senior military person, and I was fortunate that everyone on the trip managed to behave. I must admit that there were a few soldiers whose objective for the trip appeared to be consuming as much alcohol as humanly possible before they returned to the land of two beers a day. No one was there to greet us when we arrived, so we all just slunk away to our rooms to try and prepare ourselves for the challenges that tomorrow is sure to bring.

Dear Lord, please watch over everyone serving in theatre and help the next eleven and a half weeks to go by quickly. Amen!

---

13 November 1998

I had trouble getting to sleep last night. I was anxious about what the next few days would hold. While we were away, one of our Czech HIP helicopters crashed and killed all three soldiers on board. This is the third Czech helicopter to crash in the last few years – I am no longer looking forward to taking a helicopter ride anywhere in the AOR.

My 0620hrs morning run was spent within the confines of the camp because I could not find a partner to train with. What strikes me the most is how lifeless our camp seems to have become. It is almost as if someone put a vacuum in this place and sucked out all the energy. This could just be me looking at the place through tired eyes, but I think it may have more to do with the oncoming cold weather and diminishing daylight. It now gets dark here at 1700hrs, which will make it more difficult to play basketball the way we used to.

A whole lot of little things happened while I was away, so I ended up dealing with them from 0800 to 2020hrs. They included several admissions, medical repatriations, pending charges, and humanitarian aid, as well as signing invoices, seeing patients, attending meetings, and on and on. I opened my computer to find that I had seventy-three e-mails awaiting my personal attention, and I can only hope that the majority of them are no longer relevant. I found myself dealing with all these issues with a certain amount of detachment – almost as if I was a visitor who was just passing through. I imagine that this feeling will last for a few more days, and then I will be right back in the saddle. Hooah! Hooah!

I am told that Saddam Hussein is once again misbehaving in Iraq and that my brother-in-law Kevin will likely have to go over again as an AWACS (Airborne Warning and Control System) commander on what he refers to as Saddam's "Operation Deny Christmas." Kevin is convinced that Saddam does this every year at this time just to damage the morale of American troops, and he's probably correct.

I have set a number of goals for myself to achieve during the final third of my tour, and I think this will be an important way of preventing me from deteriorating into a slovenly old couch potato. The personnel in the National Command Element have started calling me "Mr. Humanitarian Aid" and have adopted these all-knowing smiles whenever the subject is raised. It seems that everyone but me was aware that humanitarian aid projects often seem to spring up out of nowhere and tend to consume whoever is dumb enough to get involved. If being dumb is the only criteria one requires to be involved, then I am definitely your man. Only seventy-three days until my replacement arrives, and only eighty-one days until I get to head home!

----

14 November 1998

This morning I was awakened by the hospital staff because a young woman had passed out in the kitchen and was unresponsive to painful stimuli for approximately four minutes. It turns out that she may have had a seizure. I advised her that she would need an EEG and an assessment by a neurologist, but to my surprise, she was not remotely interested in finding out what was wrong. I believe she is concerned that if we do find out she is having seizures, we will not continue to employ her, and for most people in this region, working for us is the best job they will ever have. From that point on, my day was an unending chain of clinical demands. I saw a fractured fifth metatarsal, an MCL (medial collateral ligament) tear, a lacerated thumb, a case of gout, an acute stress reaction and a very large lipoma (a lump of fatty tissue) that required one and a half hours to remove.

Just as the day seemed to be settling down, we were informed that a helicopter was bringing us a Czech major who was involved in a motor vehicle accident and had sustained a significant head injury. When he arrived, we discovered that he had a huge laceration on the back of his skull that went right down to the bone. The injury was so large we decided we would be best to suture him up in the operating theatre under general anaesthesia. The only problem was that his C-spine films suggested that our patient may have a fracture of his third cervical vertebra. The surgeon agreed, and so the decision was made to perform the surgery using spinal precautions. The operation took one and a half hours, and I assisted the surgeon throughout the entire procedure. This was a wonderful experience as I not only got to do some sewing, but I also got to watch our surgical team in action in our own facility. We do have very good people working here, and it's nice to be a part of this special team. When the surgery was complete, I asked the CO of the ASC if she could tell whoever rolled out the "welcome back" carpet for me that I got the message and would appreciate it if they please back off a bit. She laughed and told me that I may not believe it, but the ASC was very quiet for the entire time I was away. If things keep up the way they have been for the last two days, the staff will ask to have me sent back home just so they can get some rest.

I received my first parcel of humanitarian aid in the mail today. It was a large box of toothbrushes from the Butler Toothbrush Company. From talking to Janet last night, I understand that the officer responsible for the post office at CFB Trenton is refusing to send the huge load of medical supplies that I had bundled up and asked the 3 RCR rear party in Petawawa to mail to me. I can see that the fun and games are just getting started – humanitarian aid style. I am beginning to believe one senior medical officer whose only comment on his own humanitarian aid efforts was "Darrell, it can be very difficult to do good." Dear Lord, I sure hope that he turns out to be wrong.

15 November 1998

After a night of heavy rain I awoke to see the hills of Coralici covered with a carpet of bright white snow. I am not ready for this sudden change in the weather, and the thought of working here for eleven more weeks in the snow is a little frightening given the types of roads we must travel on. While the snow was nice to look at, it scared all the army fitness enthusiasts away from running, so I ended up enjoying another wonderful hour of my life going around in circles within the confines of our relatively small camp.

The meteorologists are predicting that a meteorite shower will bombard Coralici in the next two days and that this will likely fully disrupt our satellite communication capabilities. The bottom line for the average soldier is that it will make it difficult if not impossible to call home and speak with their loved ones. I sure hope this communication breakdown doesn't last for too long.

During today's Commander's briefing I discovered that the Multinational Division Southwest where we work covers 45 percent of Bosnia and is manned by only six thousand soldiers. This area is also home to some of the most active hot spots in Bosnia. A force of fifteen thousand soldiers covers the remaining 55 percent of the country. This hardly seems like an equitable distribution of military assets. It just goes to show how much a handful of good ole Canadians are really worth.

All our intelligence briefings emphasize that while things look to be rather calm, a great deal of nefarious activity seems to be happening below the surface. It is very likely that the criminal activity and political intimidation will continue indefinitely. We have been told that with the cold weather beginning to set in, the AOR should quiet down as citizens focus on survival rather than fighting. I sincerely hope this is true because our personnel are looking very tired.

I have spent the last three days dealing with the wide variety of issues that surfaced while I was away. I am always amazed at the number of problems that can occur when there is a large group of people working to accomplish the same goal.

It is once again late, and although I am tired, I do have a much different perspective than I had when I first returned to the Box. I will just keep chipping away at the backlog of work, and I will eventually triumph. Wish me luck!

---

16 November 1998

God came to visit me at work today, and I almost didn't recognize Him. This may be because he came to our medical facility disguised as a woman who will be turning one hundred in March 1999. She came to the gate asking to be seen by one of us so that she could get some cream for the sores on her aged face. We don't normally see civilians at the front gate unless they are very ill, because if we opened the gate to everyone seeking help, we would soon be overwhelmed. I almost sent this lady away before the medical assistants told me her story, and then it was impossible to say no. When she walked into the clinic, she had five or six obvious ulcers on her face, and it was immediately apparent that she had multiple basal and squamous cell skin cancers. On closer inspection I could see that a century of sun exposure had not been kind to her, and she had innumerable areas of severe skin damage. Undoubtedly the worst area of damage was immediately below her right eye where she had a deep ulcer probably two centimetres long and one centimetre wide. It is quite likely that this cancer has penetrated the orbit of her right eye. She told me that the sores were the result of a tree hitting her in the face a month ago, but when I consulted with her nephew, he confirmed with me that she has had her facial sores for over two years now. She had walked probably a mile to be seen and made no real complaints about her problem. All she really wanted was some cream to apply to her sores. We brought her in and cleaned up her ulcers, applied some Bactroban ointment and will see if we can find a plastic surgeon who would be willing to operate on her. The location of the ulcer under her eye, the depth of penetration and her age all combined to make her too great a risk for us to attempt anything surgical in the ASC. I sure hope we can help her.

Today was busy but manageable. Prior to today, I was beginning to think that my colleagues were disappointed that the first four months of this rotation hadn't killed me, and so they were simply going to try harder.

I contacted the 3 RCR rear party in Petawawa, and the soldier responsible for postal services informed me that all our medical aid packages were sent to Trenton – he was told that they would be placed on the next sustainment flight. I wonder if the Contingent Commander contacted the senior person in the CF postal services who may have had a little talk with the captain in charge of the postal facility in Trenton. If this is true, there should be an enormous stack of packages arriving in Coralici this week, and God will have allowed me to keep my promise to the good people of Russell. Keep your fingers crossed.

---

17 November 1998

My life was made considerably more exciting last night when I was awakened at midnight to see a Bangladeshi police officer who had injured his right shoulder in a motor vehicle accident. To add insult to injury, this was his first day of duty in Bosnia. When I reviewed his x-rays, it was apparent that the individual had not only dislocated his shoulder, but he had also sheared off the greater tuberosity of his right humerus. I had never seen this particular injury, but I knew that we had to relocate his shoulder to prevent any further damage. Despite snowing him with morphine, I was unable to get him and his muscles relaxed enough for me to relocate his shoulder. Having failed at this, I called in the Sleepy Doc, and we literally paralyzed him with a cocktail of drugs. Even after this, I really had to work at putting the humerus back in place, likely because it was trapped up under the socket of the shoulder blade. When his humerus finally slipped back into place, no one was happier than me because I was close to exhaustion from all the physical effort needed to relocate his shoulder. Follow-up films not only showed that the humerus was back in place, but also that the sheared-off greater tuberosity was right where it was supposed to be. Happy, happy!

Today was my first opportunity to see patients in the clinic we are running for the Jesuit Refugee Service. This clinic was set up for us to assess children who have been injured by the weapons of war. The first child we saw was a fourteen-year-old boy who had been hit by exploding bullets in 1995. He had a metal fragment lodged in the orbit of his right eye leaving him without vision. He had all the fingers on his left hand shot off and his right foot is now home to literally hundreds of pieces of shrapnel. We have recommended that he be seen by an eye surgeon to determine if anything can be done to restore some or all of his vision. It is difficult to look at these innocent children and realize that another human being did this to them.

The saga of the humanitarian aid continues. I was informed this morning that the post office in Trenton is now threatening not to mail any package they receive with my name on it. I can't help recalling the senior officer's warning that it sure can be hard to do good. While it upsets me to hear this kind of stupidity, I refuse to let it dull my faith that the medical supplies will get here one way or another. Stay tuned!

18 November 1998

It appears that I am not the only person who is having a hard time with this humanitarian aid issue. Cpl Holland came up with a wonderful idea for a project that she entitled "Shoeboxes for Bosnia." Her idea was to have each of the twelve hundred soldiers in Bosnia prepare a shoebox for Christmas containing items that children here could use: toothbrush, toothpaste, soap, hand towel, mittens, toys, etc. It was a good idea, but unfortunately for her it has become too good an idea. People back in Canada have gotten wind of this project and are embracing it with the same enthusiasm that the people of Russell showed towards my medical supplies project. As of now, there are more than three thousand shoeboxes in Canada waiting to be shipped overseas for Santa to deliver to Bosnian children this Christmas. However, the post office in Trenton has been advised that all packages addressed to Cpl Holland are to be put aside. These boxes will have to wait in line with all the other humanitarian aid sitting in Trenton and Petawawa awaiting an available aircraft. The wording of some of the communications suggests that the unselfish efforts of this dedicated service woman are being looked upon in a negative light. It is little wonder that many military members shy away from initiating these kinds of projects when they see one of their own treated in this way. If a general officer or their spouse had come up with the concept of Shoeboxes for Bosnia, I am certain that this story would be developing completely differently. Rank has always had its privileges and probably always will. I will do everything I can to help her get her precious cargo over here before Christmas.

We are starting to see more and more signs of stress in our soldiers. The week I returned from Canada, three guys in the same company were told by their wives that they had found someone else. I am told that at least eight guys in the Battle Group are experiencing the same marital problem. I can't imagine how hard it must be to deal with this issue when you are thousands of miles from your wife, and you aren't due to return home for another eleven more weeks. Add to this distressing situation, being away for Christmas, and you have a recipe for domestic disaster. Today we had to repatriate one of these lads because he just couldn't cope with the situation and needs to go home to try and piece his life back together. Quite often the problem appears to be that the spouse simply grows tired of being left alone and ends up finding someone else. This is a major issue because with an army as small as ours and the world as unstable as it currently is, the Canadian soldier of the future is going to be spending a great deal of time away from home. Lord, please help these soldiers because they are truly hurting and there isn't much I can do to help.

---

19 November 1998

It has become quite cold in the mornings and evenings. While this is not as pleasant as it was when it was consistently 20°C, it does have its definite advantages. It is getting too cold for the fighting factions to be out and about causing trouble. In fact, if the intelligence briefings are any indication, everyone here appears to have suddenly gone into hibernation for the winter. This sure would be nice as it will take some pressure off the Battle Group and allow our troops to relax a little.

Today was one of those "I can't believe I got all my priorities done" days. I needed this, and for the first time since my return to the theatre, I feel that I have a grip on what is going on. Our lawyer returned from his leave today with a case of pneumonia in his lungs but a rested look on his face. It was interesting to hear him say that he has returned to the theatre with a changed outlook. We laughed when I shared with him that I had the same experience and that this likely comes with operational maturity.

The struggle regarding the transportation of all the humanitarian aid back in Canada continues to give many of the people in the contingent a headache. I have decided to keep working hard on my role in this complex operation and leave the big problems up to God. I figure that if he wants this to happen, he will work out a way for Cpl Holland's and my stuff to get over here, and all I would likely accomplish would be to get in his way.

I had a chance to talk to Janet today, and it was nice to hear her voice. I miss her, the kids and the crazy cats. Nathan had his OPP Auxiliary interview last night and is confident that it went well. The interviewers asked him when he had his last physical confrontation, and his response was to ask, "On or off the ice?" The officers conducting the interview seemed to think this was quite humorous. Nathan would very much like to get into law enforcement, and I think he would do very well at it. Dear Lord, if this is where you would like my oldest son to go, please help him along this path.

The Signal Squadron was nice enough to repair my CD player that had stopped working prior to my leave. It is sure nice to once again have my nightly tunes to listen to while I am working in my office. I have worked quite hard this week, and I think I will treat myself to a movie and an early night. I am also on call tonight, so we will see what happens.

---

20 November 1998

Today was the first time we have enjoyed a snowfall of any significant volume – enough to leave the ground carpeted in white and the roads extremely slippery. I can see why one would want to keep the driving around here to a minimum during bad weather. Given the unaccustomed quiet that has suddenly fallen upon the AOR, I have decided that the best way to ensure peace in Bosnia would be to have snow, cold temperatures and short days year-round. I may be dreaming, but this seems to be the only thing keeping the opposing sides from going at each other's throats.

My run this morning was very cold, and when it was finally over, I was rewarded with an even colder shower. I have taken to lathering up my body before I go into the shower to reduce the amount of time I must suffer through my daily polar dip. It wouldn't surprise me to find out that the Army would prefer us to have cold showers because hot water would open our pores and give weakness an opportunity to seep into our bodies. Hooah! Hooah!

I have just found out that the majority of the medical team that we replaced here in Bosnia is now in Honduras helping out with the disaster that occurred there. The medical team will likely be in Honduras for the next two months. These people were deployed because they are designated as part of the Disaster Assistance Response Team (DART). This team used to be called the Fast Action Response Team or FART – no joke! I can just imagine the conversations that must have taken place at the headquarters level whenever a disaster occurred:

"Tell me, General Nuisance, what capability does the Department of National Defence have to ensure that we are able to rapidly respond to emergencies around the world?"

"Well, when such situations occur the Surgeon General will respond by dispatching a good FART."

I imagine it was hard to get any respect when you told people that you served with the FART. I am also left wondering who was dumb enough to come up with this acronym. What is even more concerning is that whoever it was, they probably got promoted for it.

21 November 1998

Another Saturday night in Stalag Coralici, and I miss my family. Being here is OK, but nothing can replace sharing ordinary moments with your loved ones.

It snowed a great deal today, and as a result, there has been very little movement in the AOR. The only traffic permitted is that deemed to be operationally essential. It is also very cold at the moment, and this could make for a long couple of months in the Box.

Today I had the opportunity to discuss Cpl Holland's Shoebox for Bosnia project with the Contingent Commander. As I suspected, he was not told the entire story. I also explained to him that I thought her efforts merited a commendation and not the kick in the ass she has been getting from the Battle Group. He agreed with me and subsequently discussed this issue with the acting Battle Group Commander and Cpl Holland. I hope that this helps her achieve her goal of delivering all the donated gifts to the children in our AOR.

The mail was dropped off this evening, and out of curiosity I checked to see if I had been sent anything. To my utter amazement, I had eighteen packages delivered and three of them contained medications that we can use in the ambulantas this coming week. They also delivered fifteen packages to Cpl Holland. Thank you, Lord! Please keep the packages coming!

Today one of our medical assistants reported to work feeling quite unwell. This is a fellow who never gets ill and teases all the ill or injured soldiers who come in to be seen that they are just weak. Today was payback time for the staff. When we found that he was under the weather, we were like pit bulls on a pork chop and decided to treat him to a bit of his own medicine. I sent him to his room to get some sleep, and while he was there, we stuck a sign on the door which read "Danger, weakness zone." I was also tempted to offer him new miracle pill called Triactin. If he asked me what this drug is supposed to do, I would smile and say, "Try actin' like a man!" He seems to be a tad bit humbler than he was several days ago.

The Mess has started serving us a dessert that consists basically of pink foam. I really don't care for the taste of it, but to justify my not eating it I have been telling the lads that if I were to eat pink, I would basically be ingesting weakness and I would soon find myself wanting to "go army." We sure wouldn't want that to happen now, would we? While I greatly respect all that the army is doing here in Bosnia, I simply can't resist the opportunity to get in a dig or two. Good night free world.

22 November 1998

The snow continues to fall, and the roads are so difficult to travel on that the Battle Group has ceased doing any patrols whatsoever. This restriction has resulted in slowing down the entire pace of life in our camp. I certainly don't mind, and quite frankly, I think most of the people in theatre were ready for the change of pace.

The circuit breaker in our chapel blew when we tried to plug in a second heater this morning. We never did get things working again, and so the six of us in the congregation huddled together to try and stay warm during Mass. That was definitely the coldest Mass I have ever had the privilege of attending.

This morning's run was difficult as the roads had not been plowed, and in the hills, we were encountering snow drifts higher than our knees. Training through the next few months will be a challenge to say the least.

Cpl Holland and I received good news today, in that the Army could not deliver some Iltis vehicles to Trenton in time to be flown over here. This should mean that there are two empty Hercules aircraft that are available to carry the humanitarian aid. I am praying that they will stuff both aircraft with the multitude of Shoeboxes for Bosnia that are currently being stored in Trenton. Wouldn't that be a miracle?

This afternoon I decided to take some time for myself and spent it working on our family letters. From the time we were first married, every Christmas season, I prepare a light-hearted record of what happened in our family that year. These letters eventually became known as the Menard Family Letters. Reading these letters provided me with an amazing trip down memory lane. Going over the letters allowed me to go back to the years when the kids were youngsters and relive some of the highlights of our life together. Many of these little gems might have been lost in the mist of time if we had never taken the

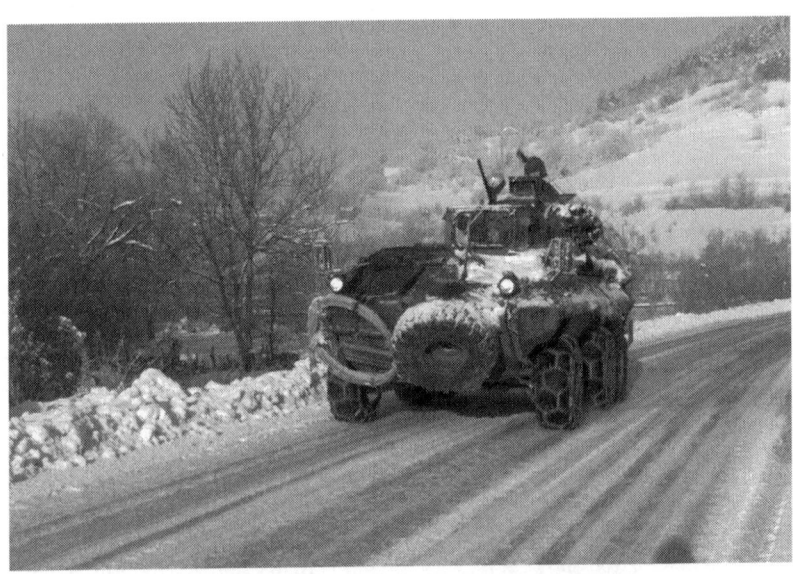

One of the countless patrols performed by Canadian soldiers during our deployment. Chains were placed on the tires to make it safer to travel on Bosnia's slippery winter roads.

time to record them. I am so glad that Janet and I had the smarts to save these letters because I am certain they will become increasingly precious to us as time goes by. Only ten more weeks till we get to head home for good. Yeah!

---

23 November 1998

I survived yet another day filled with all kinds of demands. These hectic days sure help time fly, but they do get to be somewhat frustrating especially when you are trying to simultaneously focus your attention on a number of different priorities. While I was on my R&R, I had the shoemaker put a thick set of Vibram soles on both pairs of my combat boots. Not only are the boots significantly more comfortable, but they also make me much taller. The soldiers have begun referring to them as my Frankenstein boots, and I think that deep down they are jealous they don't have a set of their own. We were graced with a visit from the new Deputy Chief of the Defence Staff this morning, but no one appeared to be overly excited. People here are quite tired of functioning as the entertainment crew for VIPs. The Surgeon General's visit was one of the few that I can honestly say was useful, and perhaps this is because I have a medical bias.

For lunch today, I decided to have the soup du jour and a tuna fish sandwich. When I sat down to eat, I commented to one of my colleagues that the soup was very thick today. As I merrily ate away, I couldn't help but notice that the people around me had their meat loaf topped with a sauce that bore a remarkable resemblance to the soup I was eating. It wasn't until someone sat down beside me with a bowl of beef soup that I realized I was eating a gigantic bowl of meat loaf sauce. It was pretty good, and I finished it off feeling full and a great deal dumber than when I started the day.

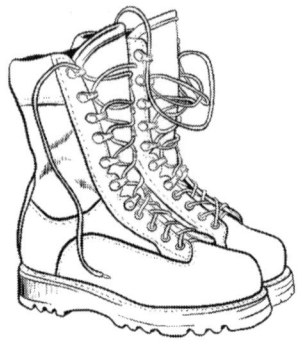

My Frankenstein combat boots

The CAF can be a frustrating place to work at times, especially when you see people like Cpl Holland, who show outstanding initiative, being punished instead of congratulated. A soldier I was talking to summed up this tendency eloquently by saying, "In our organization, a pat on the back is often just reconnaissance for where to insert the blade." Regrettably, I am starting to believe there may be a lot of truth to what he said.

Folks in the "head shed" are still investigating the death of the young soldier who was electrocuted, and fingers are pointing towards individuals who the troops feel could have prevented this tragic accident. I am sure we will be seeing soldiers coming for help to deal with the stress associated with all of this.

---

24 November 1998

The temperature has warmed significantly today, and all the nice white snow that we were blessed with has turned to wet, brown slush.

In this type of weather, the nice thing about my new combat boots is that my sole is so high that my boots never get wet. Who says the Air Force can't teach the Army a few tricks?

You know you have been in theatre too long when the troops start referring to the one-room kit shop as "the mall." This is really the only place we can go Christmas shopping, and while the staff are doing their best, most of the stuff they have brought in for gifts is really tacky. One item that pretty much says it all is a T-shirt with the inscription: "My father went to Bosnia and all he got me was this lousy T-shirt." Could you imagine anyone not longing to have a wardrobe full of these in a variety of inspiring colours? It is unfortunate but I would prefer to wait until I am home to get my loved ones something nice for Christmas.

This morning, we operated on a young man who had the misfortune of being blown up by a land mine several years ago. The explosion took off most of his left leg and half of his right lower leg. Since his tragic accident, he has had to endure five major operations to allow him to be able to walk with a prosthesis on his left leg. Even after all this, his left fibula extends well below his left tibia, and this makes it very painful to wear his prosthesis. Our surgeon felt that it would take about fifteen minutes to open his stump, trim back the fibula and close the wound. Unfortunately, the day did not go as planned. To begin with, the patient ate breakfast, and then he decided he did not want a general anaesthetic. Our anaesthetist skilfully performed an epidural nerve block, and while it took a while to take effect, we were ready to go by 1145hrs. Everything was going well until it was time to cut the dissected end of the fibula. This procedure had to be done blindly, and during the process we nicked the popliteal artery. With a blood vessel this big, the first indication of a problem is a large gush of blood. We got just that, and then spent the next ninety minutes trying to get the wound to stop bleeding. Ultimately, things looked great, but we sure had to work hard for that result. I sincerely hope that what we did for this young man will allow him to function better for the rest of his life.

25 November 1998

Only one month left until Christmas, and I wish I could spend it in the arms of my loved ones, enjoying their laughs, smiles and engaging conversation. It will be a hard time of year for everyone here and for their families back home. I cannot imagine how hard it must be for young children who do not understand why daddy or mommy can't be there to open presents with them.

The Can Con show will soon be here to entertain the troops. These performances are a lot like the Bob Hope shows the Americans used to have in Vietnam. They have posters up all over the camp and someone modified a number of the posters located in high traffic areas. The culprit added a picture of the camp commandant and indicated that he would be putting on an exhibition of exotic dancing. I thought it was very funny, but I suspect the camp commandant didn't appreciate the humour, as I saw him in the Mess tearing all the posters down and throwing them in the garbage. It's too bad he can't take a joke.

Today was clinically busy and this sure helps to make the day go by quickly. I tried out an ophthalmic cautery pen on a cherry angioma located on a soldier's face and it worked fantastically. We have no hyfrecator unit here in theatre and I think these little pens will serve as an excellent substitute.

I had an opportunity to talk to Nathan tonight, and I could hear the worry in his voice. He has had a series of incapacitating headaches recently and now has a slightly dilated right pupil and ringing in his right ear. He was given a CT scan that was interpreted as normal – in other words, no tumour. However, an aneurysm or an arteriovenous malformation would not show up on a CT scan. To be identified, these two conditions will require an arteriogram. Nathan will meet the neurologist tomorrow and is very anxious to know what the next steps will be. It is times like this that make it very hard to be so far away from someone you care about. No matter what you say over the phone, it will never replace the love and caring you can transmit with a warm hug.

The ASC staff watched a movie entitled City of Angels this evening. It certainly makes a person think about what is really important in life, and for me that is definitely my family. Lord, please look after my loved ones, and as a special prayer, please reach out your hand and keep my eldest child safe.

---

26 November 1998

Only sixty-eight days till I get to go home – I am pretty sure I am not the only one who is counting.

This morning, I finally discovered why I have been so clinically busy lately. It appears that the soldiers have heard that Doc Menard is pretty "switched on" when it comes to sports injuries and the lads are coming in from all over wanting to have their aches and pains examined. This is kind of a win-win situation in that they get their problems looked at, and I get an opportunity to practise my craft.

The weather has remained warm, which means that the roads are once again becoming decent places to run. This is a good thing because all the running enthusiasts in the contingent really are aching for the opportunity to get in a good workout.

I enjoy watching figure skating and somehow the lads have found out that I'm huge fan of Katarina Witt. She was a two-time Olympic champion and is considered one of the greatest singles figure skaters of all time. The guys appear to be experiencing fiendish delight taking turns telling me they have a copy of Playboy's Christmas issue in which there is a very revealing article on Miss Witt and her many assets. I am certain the article is merely a documentary of her outstanding athletic achievements. Anyway, they all seem to be real sports fans and are now wondering what I have to trade for this valuable piece of Pulitzer Prize winning literature. I don't suppose my copy of James Herriot's Vet in Harness will give me much bargaining power.

Nathan had his appointment with the neurologist today, and in typical sensitive medical consultant fashion he informed Nathan that if he had had an aneurysm, they wouldn't be having this conversation because Nathan would already be dead. Despite his bluntness, the neurologist made Nathan's day and took a big load of worry off Janet and me.

The humanitarian aid saga continues, and we will be having a big pow wow about it tomorrow morning. It appears that the response to Cpl Holland's idea has been so good that it may have overwhelmed our ability to store and distribute the shoeboxes even if a civilian carrier were to give us a helping hand. This is causing the logistics folks to lose sleep at night.

I have heard concerning rumours about the contingent that is coming in to replace us. They apparently aren't interested in doing any humanitarian aid. Unbelieveable! One of the doctors scheduled to deploy has been deemed medically unfit because he cannot carry a rucksack. His alternative cannot come because he has asthma and will be released in July '99. The surgeon who is scheduled to replace our current surgeon is reported to be so out of shape he can barely make it up a flight of stairs, and even though he failed all his fitness testing they are still planning to send him into theatre. If he were an infantry soldier, he would be shown the door and told not to come back. This is the kind of double standard that the troops get upset about and I can't blame them. It also embarrasses me that we demand that our troops be fit, but not some of our specialized medical personnel. With stuff like this going on, I am not surprised to hear that the morale in the CAF is at an all-time low.

27 November 1998

We had the Commander's conference this morning, and a meeting on humanitarian aid was supposed to follow. At the conclusion of the conference, nothing had been mentioned referencing the meeting's location, so I asked about it, and two young captains quickly responded that the meeting had been cancelled. I must have had a very puzzled look on my face because the Commander invited me to meet with him privately. When we got behind closed doors, I informed him how large the Shoebox project had become and that, while he never asked for this project to be undertaken, I could see no way for the contingent to avoid becoming involved. I even showed him an article from the *Ottawa Citizen* newspaper with a picture of the Minister of National Defence holding a Christmas Shoebox and proclaiming how much he was looking forward to hand-delivering some shoeboxes to children on his upcoming visit to Bosnia. I also informed him that if DND didn't get on the bandwagon soon, we would be asked some very embarrassing questions by important people who would be demanding answers. I showed him Cpl Holland's scrapbook with all the newspaper stories and the faxes from all over Canada. Something must have gone right during our brief interaction because thirty minutes after we talked, he sent out an e-mail to everyone who is anyone in the contingent indicating the importance of Cpl Holland's project and that "we" will do everything we can to ensure it's a success. He officially named the project "OP SHOEBOX." We will have a big meeting tomorrow morning to form a project team with people from all the major units needed to handle the various aspects of delivering these gifts into the hands of disadvantaged Bosnian children. The real irony is that one of the young captains who cut me off and told the Commander that the humanitarian aid meeting was cancelled ended up being appointed to coordinate the project for the CCSFOR HQ. I sure hope that this works out for the better.

I received a letter today that was addressed to "Any Canadian Soldier." It was written by a fourteen-year-old girl in Ontario. It was moving to read that she was very proud of all that we are doing and wondered how we handled being separated from our families for such long periods. I took the time to write her back and thank her for her kind words of encouragement. It is nice to know that there are young Canadians who are sensitive enough to think about peacekeepers at Christmas time. She asked why the people of the world can't live in peace. The only thing I could tell her was that I shared her concern and wished I knew the answer.

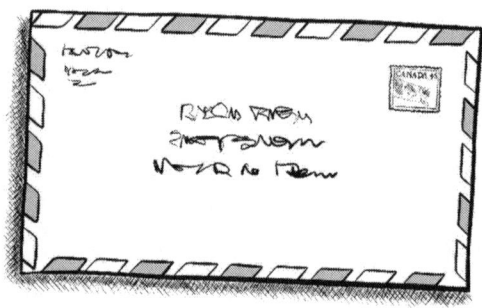

Christmas letter addressed to any Canadian Soldier

---

28 November 1998

This morning's meeting for Operation Shoebox was chaired by the Contingent Commander and went very well. He emphasized for every-one in attendance that this was a great idea and that the soldiers in CCSFOR were being afforded a great privilege by generous Canadians who were entrusting us with the responsibility of hand-delivering their gifts to needy Bosnian children. It is amazing how having the colonel on board has changed everyone's attitude towards this project. Everyone has gone from being negative to being fully supportive within a mere twenty-four-hour period. I have not endeared myself to the young captains, but something valuable is being accomplished and this isn't a popularity contest.

One of our staff was ill this afternoon, and when he began to feel better, we decided to have some fun with him. While he was resting on the ward, I sent another member of the staff to give him a fleet enema to help purge the weakness from him. For the briefest moment he thought we were serious, and this made it all worthwhile. We topped off our mischief by having the Padre show up in full garb to give him his last rights. Neither of them could stop laughing long enough for us to get a quality photo. Life is too short not to have some fun, even when you are working in a theatre of operations.

Refugees from Kosovo have elected to settle in one of the most unstable areas in our AOR. The citizens in this area are primarily Croatian, and this could cause problems as we have been told that the only thing that Croatians hate more than Serbs is Kosovars. It will be interesting to see if this sparks a new round of limited violence.

Winding roads, slippery surfaces and the totally insane driving habits of the locals have significantly increased the rate of accidents that the contingent is experiencing. This week there were five motor vehicle accidents and only one of them was determined to be a Canadian soldier's fault. Thank goodness no one was seriously injured. Let's hope that this luck continues while we are here.

Two weapons holding areas were broken into this week and the thieves made off with sixty machine guns and other assorted weapons. This robbery might increase the fun and games that occur in our AOR. This seems to me to be a relatively easy way to acquire some serious firepower, and I predict that we will see an increase in this kind of misbehaviour.

---

29 November 1998

It has now been nearly two weeks since the sun has shone on the hills of Coralici, which is a bit depressing for everyone. I shouldn't complain – much of the snow has melted and the temperatures are warmer than they were ten days ago.

This evening, I was examining a female patient who was having some visual disturbances likely related to her recurrent migraine headaches. When I asked how she was doing, she informed me that whenever she focused on my face it made her very nauseated. I told her not to worry because many women who look me experience the same feeling. We eventually decided to start an IV on her. The female medical assistant who was helping me, knew the patient had very poor veins and that it would likely be a difficult IV to start. Instead of saying this, she stated that the woman has always been a "hard poke"! Thanks to my extensive training in political correctitude, I didn't jump on this line, but I really wanted to.

Cpl Holland and I discovered today that the new buzzword in the contingent is "Op Shoebox." Apparently if we are having trouble getting anything done, all we have to do is tell the people who are being difficult that this is for Op Shoebox and all doors will open. This is a far cry from forty-eight hours prior when the mere mention of humanitarian aid was likely to get you thrown out of someone's office. I am told that the Commander has generated an Op Order (Operations Order) for Op Shoebox and informed the Chief of the Defence Staff about what is happening. This makes the entire project very official and should generate considerable interest in providing it with full operational support. When all the dust finally settles, I sincerely hope that every needy child in Bosnia gets a shoebox delivered to them by a smiling Canadian soldier. I also pray that the local medical facilities receive some useful supplies to help them care for those who cannot afford to go anywhere else.

I found out today that Rebecca's basketball team won the Eastern Ontario High School Basketball Championships and that they will be competing in the Ontario championships next week. This is an incredible achievement considering how small her school is. I would give my eye teeth to be able to sit and enjoy watching the girls compete at such a big event. Missing these once-in-a-lifetime events hurts when you are stuck here in the Box.

---

30 November 1998

Yet another fun-filled day here in theatre, and as evening draws to a close, I hope that all the work we are doing in Bosnia turns out to be worthwhile. Between seeing patients and dealing with my medical advisor responsibilities, Op Shoebox and my own projects, I definitely don't find myself suffering from boredom.

I ended up admitting a patient with severe pain behind her right eye, and although she does have a history of migraine headaches, the location of this discomfort did not match anything she had ever experienced before. I was convinced it was a simple migraine until I was informed that nothing she has been given in the past has helped during an intense episode – just the kind of thing you want to hear from a patient whose head feels like it is about to explode. Being conservative by nature, I started her off on a low dose of chlorpromazine. After an hour without a response, I doubled the dose and basically knocked the patient out. When she awoke four or five hours later, she felt hungover, but her pain was gone. Thanks for the help, Lord!

Sean Upton of the CBC has been trying to get through to me to follow up on the humanitarian aid efforts from Russell, and this evening we finally managed to connect. He ended up doing an interview with Cpl Holland and me on Op Shoebox, and we discussed how our efforts to get the humanitarian aid from Canada to Bosnia were going. The interview seemed to go well, and Cpl Holland and I were both careful to sound as positive as possible. Little would have been accomplished by telling the press how hard we were having to push to try and get our humanitarian aid over here before Christmas. If all goes well, this interview will be heard by the right set of ears and Op Shoebox will be given another set of helping hands or two. If this effort fails, it sure won't be for lack of trying.

My parents sent me another box of gifts, and this one contained a variety of beautiful cloths for use on the altars in the various chapels in theatre. They will look very nice during Christmas Mass.

I talked to Janet this afternoon – I sure do miss her and the children. I even miss our mangy, flea-bitten, butt-sniffing, rear end-licking cats. Dear Lord, please watch over my loved ones and help all our Canadian soldiers to return home safely. Amen.

December 1998

1 December 1998

One more month down and two more to go. It snowed again this evening, and it is absolutely beautiful outside. It would be nice to share a night like this with my family.

The Divisional Surgeon and two of his staff dropped in for a friendly visit this morning. They flew over in one of our Griffon helicopters, and it was the first time one of our birds landed in Coralici. We gave them a tour of our medical facilities and spent a fair bit of time discussing issues relevant to the multinational provision of health care in Bosnia. While we were touring the laboratory, we had them stop and look at a microscope slide with a positive swab for gonorrhea. The slide contained pink and black tissue, and I told them to ignore the black substances because they were tonsillar tissues. When they asked why we would have tonsillar tissue on a penile swab, I informed them that our techs are instructed to stick the penile swabs as high up as possible. Hooah! You don't have to be terribly creative to imagine how gonorrhea might get onto a soldier's tonsillar tissue.

It is nice to have our own choppers in theatre, but they are such temperamental pieces of equipment that they have been unable to fly most of the time here because of the poor weather. Today was a classic example of this. As soon as it began to snow, we knew that our British guests would be unable to fly back home. This was confirmed by the Flight Safety Control Centre, so we arranged for them to spend the night with us. This put a crimp in everyone's plans. While they were settling into their rooms, I went to examine a patient who turned out to be one of our liaison officers working at the same base as our guests. It just so happened that he was heading back there shortly and had just enough room in his Land Rover to accommodate them. The Brits jumped at the chance because the forecasted weather could have seen them stuck in Stalag Coralici for a very long time.

During the day, the radiology tech asked to talk to me privately in the x-ray suite. Assuming only medical staff would be in the ASC, when our discussion was over, I exited the office pretending to be pulling my pants back up and thanking him for the wonderful oral discussion. When I turned to the left, however, I noticed a female warrant officer waiting to have an x-ray taken. I burst out laughing and told her that we really didn't have that close of a working relationship. I'm not entirely sure that she believed me. Coincidently, I was later informed that I will be seeing her as a patient tomorrow. This should be interesting.

It would appear that sometime during the day a naughty person switched the major's slip ons on my Gore-Tex jacket and replaced them with those of a corporal. I must have walked around for half the day before someone pointed out my dress code problem. Using my incredible detective skills, I have ferreted out the culprit's identity and will seek my retribution when my victim least expects it.

––––––––––––––

2 December 1998

We continue to see young soldiers who are picking up sexually transmitted diseases in Budapest. The troops have started referring to this fun town as "Bootie-Fest." One of the brothels there, Captain Jacks, caters only to Canadian soldiers. The expression being used in the camp these days is "First you meet Captain Jack, and then you meet Major Menard." I asked our latest victim if he had noted anything unusual about the woman who shared her infection with him. He looked at me with absolute sincerity and said, "No! She smelled great! And tasted even better." Everyone in the medical inspection room burst out laughing and it took some time for us to regain our professional composure. I guarantee that even if I live to be one hundred, I will never forget that line. For the remainer of our deployment, this soldier's innocent response became a popular mantra for the medical team – especially at mealtime. I don't know what it will take to get our soldiers to realize the risks they are taking when they have unprotected sex in these houses of ill repute.

The Can Con troop arrived in camp to put on an evening show for all the soldiers in Coralici, and you can feel the excitement in the air. Every Christmas, these folks travel all over the world to provide a little good ole Canadian entertainment to our soldiers. They use a time-tested formula consisting of girls, comedy, girls, music, girls, dancing, girls and lastly more girls. The soldiers cleared out our large vehicle mainte-nance bay and set up a stage with seating for 250 people.

The production was very professional and yet still managed to maintain a warm and friendly atmosphere. The comedians were hilarious, and they tailored their jokes to match our current living situation. They had a very good backup band and several very good singers. One of the country and western singers currently has a num-ber of songs that are in the top ten on the charts – I believe his name is Jamie Warren. He really does have a beautiful voice. There were six dancing girls and everything they wore was skimpy – much to the delight of every male soldier in the house (except for me of course – I chastely spent the moments they were on stage in pious reflection). Every time they came on stage the lads went wild and you could al-most feel the testosterone in the air.

The show lasted a total of two and a half hours, and the cast con-cluded by singing, "We Wish You a Merry Christmas." This choked me up a bit because it sure brought home the fact that none of us will be spending Christmas with our families. Several of the entertainers took the opportunity to thank us for honourably representing our country and making a real contribution towards world peace. This meant a great deal to me and quite likely to many of the soldiers in the audience.

3 December 1998

We said goodbye to the Can Con troop this morning. This evening, they will be putting on their last show for our soldiers in VK. Everyone that I talked to enjoyed the performances. The stage crew had a meet-and-greet last night, and then the band held a jam session in the Junior Ranks' Mess until 0400hrs. They really did put a little sparkle in our otherwise routine lives.

While we were enjoying the Can Con show, SFOR troops snatched another person wanted for war crimes in Bosnia. This person turned out to be the general in command of all of 5th Corps — one of the warring faction's major military units. He was quickly taken to The Hague where he will stand trial for his crimes against the citizens of Bosnia. In response, 5th Corps has been put on alert, and we may see some reprisals. This is just what you want to see happen during the Christmas season.

The CAF just announced that it will be sending ten medical per-sonnel to work with the French in Macedonia. While I am not certain what their mission will be, it is likely related in some way to the con-flict in Kosovo.

Captain Edora returns to camp tonight, and once again my life here will change significantly. While I am happy to have my running buddy back, I am also somewhat disappointed because I will no longer be doing the majority of the patient care for the camp. On the upside, I will now have some freedom to travel to see a few of the units I have yet to visit, such as Aviano (Italy) and Tuzla. I will also have a great deal more time available to do fun things such as paperwork, boot polishing, parade drill, weapons training and rucksack marches. Hooah!

At all the meetings I now attend, there is a prevailing feeling that everyone here is very tired. I know that I am. We have all worked an enormous number of hours, and a person can only do that for so long before you start to feel beat up. On the positive side, people in the camp are starting to get to know each other very well, and I enjoy wandering around saying hello to patients and acquaintances alike. Despite this increasing sense of familiarity with the personnel around me, I remain at my core a very private person, and I miss the intimacy of my family. It would be so very nice to spend this evening in the arms of my wife, telling her how much I love her. Unfortunately, this will have to wait awhile.

---

4 December 1998

God blessed Coralici with a heavy snowfall, but this evening it began to rain. If the temperature drops, it could make life around here very interesting. The roads were so bad today that only operationally essential driving was permitted.

On my morning run, I was joined by two groups of young children who simply wanted to hold hands and run with a crazy Canadian soldier. They picked the right guy.

Captain Edora returned from his leave late last night. The lads had short-sheeted his bed and taped a picture from Playgirl magazine above his head. Nothing like having the red carpet rolled out for you – army style. The Chief of the Air Staff, LGen Kinsman, paid us a visit today. Although I wasn't invited to be part of the head table, he recognized me and called me over to say hello. While we were shaking hands, the Battle Group Commander kindly reminded me that I had been given specific instructions: when we have guests, I am not allowed to eat in the same room as them. I promised to hide behind another officer so that I wouldn't embarrass anyone with my barbaric eating habits.

I learned a new army medical term this week. A patient that I was examining had been suffering from constipation but finally managed to have a painful bowel movement. When I asked him why he was here to see me, he told me that he had experienced a "hard extraction." In a traditional army sense, this is a term used to describe a situation in which it is difficult to remove a spent casing from a weapon. The analogy of applying this to passing a stubborn bowel movement works for me (and is oddly poetic for an army guy).

Every week a different unit gets to select the evening movies that will be played at the Mess. The army fellas absolutely dread "ASC week" because that is when all the feel-good movies get played. They simply will not come to the Mess for fear that watching a sensitive movie will somehow give weakness a foothold in their bodies. For most grunts, their idea of a tear-jerking, romantic movie is Rambo III.

This afternoon we were contacted by the United Nations High Commissioner for Refugees (UNHCR) whose job it is to look after formerly displaced citizens returning to their homes in Bosnia. Members of their staff had visited a woman who lives about two and a half hours from here in a remote area in which there is a border dispute. Apparently, she had run out of her medications, and they wanted us to go and pick her up and take her to the hospital in Bihac. As nice as this would be to do, the BG refused to put a group of soldiers at risk for someone who does not appear to be critically ill. The first question that we asked the UNHCR was why they didn't put her in their vehicle and bring her to the hospital themselves if they were that concerned about her. Unfortunately, common sense does not appear to be all that common even in the UNHCR.

---

5 December 1998

We awoke to nearly a foot of fresh snow this morning, and the sun shone brightly for the first time in twenty-three days. It would have been an ideal day for flying around in the hills on a pair of cross-country skis – except for the ever-present risk of land mines.

Once again, all the meetings scheduled for today were cancelled – what a blessing! This included our visit to a family with eight children whose entire living space is estimated to be no more than one hundred square feet. We are told this family is in need of many things and one of the platoons appears to have adopted them. I hope that we can somehow make their lives a little better. I spent the majority of the day working on administrative tasks that I had left unattended while Captain Edora was away. Although these things do need to get done, they somehow just don't seem to be nearly as important as taking care of our patients.

The medical donations from the American medical staff in Zagreb were finally delivered this afternoon. Our American colleagues ended up sending ten boxes packed with all kinds of useful medications and supplies. The mail also arrived today, and I found this to be a very frustrating experience. There are soldiers receiving a wide variety of humanitarian donations, while Cpl Holland and I cannot seem to get our stuff onto a plane headed to Bosnia. One young captain received over twenty boxes of materials. I need to remind myself that these people are also having important donations sent over to Bosnia. Why should my supplies take precedence over anyone else's? My faith in God must be very weak these days because I can't help but worry that Op Shoebox will not be assigned a military aircraft, and we will not get the humanitarian aid delivered before Christmas. I feel very impotent because there doesn't seem to be a great deal more that I can do at this point. Please Lord, we sure could use your help getting Op Shoebox off the ground – literally.

---

6 December 1998

Another day and another adventure here in theatre. Yesterday was very warm, and all our snow turned into a slushy mess, only to freeze solid again overnight. As a result, almost all our running routes have been rendered unusable. From here on in, we may be doing a great deal of running up and down the same boring road or on an equally boring treadmill. This will get old very quickly.

After church today, several of us packed up a bunch of the humanitarian aid that Canadians have sent to us and went for a long ride in search of the family that our patrols claim is very poor and in desperate need of help. When we were about three hundred metres away from their home, the Bison we were driving in slid off the road, and half of the vehicle got stuck in the ditch. There was no way we were getting out on our own. Why does this seem to happen to me whenever I travel anywhere here in this war torn country? We ended up walking to their home, and what we witnessed was a distressing level of poverty in the midst of an otherwise nice village. The family claims that they have received no support from the community because they are DNZ supporters, and the majority of the village residents are SDA party members. The rundown shack in which they live has multiple rooms but only one of them is heated. This room is approximately ten feet by twelve feet, and it is where seven children, a father and a mother who is nine months pregnant, live and sleep. The small oven that they use to cook and heat their living space is beginning to fall apart and will soon become a serious fire hazard. Prior to our arrival, they were nearly out of food. They have very few blankets and no proper winter footwear. The dad told us that he worked for six months this summer in Croatia, but when he was done, his employer refused to pay him. Prior to the war, they were starting to build a new house, but during the war years people came and stole all their building materials. Although the mom is only thirty-seven, she looks considerably older. The good news is that her pregnancy is going very well, and her main concern is how she will pay the fees for delivering her baby in the local hospital. Her children have all been healthy and look quite well.

With our Bison stuck in the ditch, we ended up humping our supplies to them. This took quite a while. We brought them twenty-five

kilograms of flour, eight large bottles of cooking oil, a large bag of pota-
toes, a bag of carrots, chocolate bars, pudding cups, cookies, cheese dips,
apples, oranges, boxes of winter clothing, blankets, toys and some of
Cpl Holland's famous Christmas shoeboxes. I have recommended to the
BG that these people be plugged into a local support agency. If necessary,
I will find some money to pay for the mother's delivery and hospital fees.
Three hours later, our extraction vehicle arrived and carefully pulled
our vehicle from the ditch. We then headed home to a supper the likes
of which the family we just left have not seen in many years. Thank you,
Lord, for all that you have given me and all that you have not.

7 December 1998

Man, is it ever getting cold here in the early mornings! This morning, the air temperature felt like minus 20°C. This is bad enough but
knowing that the folks back home are experiencing near tropical
weather doesn't help matters. These temperatures sure do separate
the men from the boys – if this distinction were based solely on who
is out running in the mornings, there don't appear to be many men
left in Stalag Coralici.

I have started compiling a list of army medical terms, and the term
of the day is "malingerer." According to the dictionary definition, a
malingerer is "a person who pretends or exaggerates incapacity or illness to avoid duty or work," (Merriam-Webster Dictionary) but in the
army it appears to mean "anyone who shows up to be seen at the unit
medical station regardless of how ill they happen to be." Based on my
experience here in theatre, this isn't all that far from the truth.

We currently have personnel working at the top of several mountains where they operate and maintain radio re-broadcasting sites.
These places have been under snow for a long time now, and the only

way to get supplies up to them is to use a bulldozer to clear the road so that other vehicles can make it up the mountain trails. Today our bulldozer rolled off the side of the mountain and is upside down in a huge snowbank. The driver was lucky to walk away with only minor acid burns from the damaged battery located under the seat. But for the grace of God, this could very easily have been our third death this tour and would have devastated everyone's morale. The roads have become increasingly dangerous to be on, so people here are travelling less and less.

This evening, I received very disturbing news from one of my best friends, Wayne Lee. Apparently, his son Robin was stabbed in the abdomen outside a bar in Hull, Quebec. The knife missed his aorta and several other important structures by an inch. He is stable and should recover completely thanks to the miracle of modern medicine. The assailant's motivation for the stabbing apparently was to display his anger at the fact that his girlfriend seemed to be paying more attention to Robin than to him. The tragedy is that this idiot will probably get away with a slap on the wrist and not the jail sentence he so richly deserves.

The CO of the ASC and I have both noticed an obvious coolness from the CO of the Battle Group. I certainly hope that it has nothing to do with the issue of humanitarian aid, but I suspect that it very well may. Personally, I don't care how the BG leadership feels about me. I just hope it does not interfere with our ability to continue helping Bosnians in need.

---

8 December 1998

This morning was the coldest day we have yet encountered, and once again I was treated to an ice-cold shower after my morning workout. It took me until 0930hrs to finally thaw out. I had a chance to see my first case of confirmed gonococcal pharyngitis today. I am certain this young man would have thought twice about having a sexual encounter if he had known the price he would be paying after.

Operation Shoebox had a monumental day today. It started off with someone informing us of the Minister of National Defence's announcement: he will be coming to Bosnia, and he wants the staff here to schedule him in on the 19th of December to present some Bosnian children with shoeboxes. Apparently, he made the front cover of a national newspaper helping a reserve unit package up shoeboxes to send to us. The paper quotes him as saying, "This is a great idea." You should see the folks around here starting to move on things. I really have no burning desire to meet the Minister, but I do hope his trip to Bosnia and his interest in Op Shoebox will help us get the transport aircraft we require.

As unbelievable as this may sound, eight hours later I received a message from the Commander indicating that DND has somehow found an airbus to carry all our supplies over and that it will depart Canada on the 12th of December. This is marvelous, stupendous, terrific, incredible, wonderful and about bloody time! This flight and the space available on the other flights coming over should allow us to get all the outstanding humanitarian aid from Canada. This includes between five and six thousand shoeboxes, the winter clothing from Russell and all our medical supplies – not to mention all the other items, some of which have been awaiting delivery for nearly a year. The icing on the cake is that the fella who coordinates the pickup and delivery of the humanitarian aid in Ottawa happens to be an old running buddy of mine, and if he can't help Janet get the boxes of clothing from our garage to Trenton, then no one can. Thank you, Lord, for your help in this enormous effort. A lot of us over here have been trying to do your will, and you sure came through for us in a big-time way. God is good!

9 December 1998

Only fifty-five more sleeps till I get to leave this frozen and highly dysfunctional place forever! It was once again extremely cold this morning. The heating systems in all our rooms, offices and messes are inadequate for dealing with these temperatures, and that sure makes living here a lot less fun. Some of the folks I know are sleeping with their toques and gloves on because their rooms are so cold at night. The dining hall is never warm enough to be comfortable, and many people are eating their meals with their Gor-Tex parkas on. I am looking forward to a break in this cold front so that we can stop spending all day huddled up inside.

This morning, I went to the town of Bihac to do a whole bunch of errands. I ended up dropping off blood for the Bihac hospital's blood bank. We visited the psychiatric facility that the boys in Oscar Company are renovating. The OR team was working today so I also paid them a visit. If a Canadian low-income housing project were in the same state as their surgical centre, it would be closed down until further notice: there are broken windows everywhere, the walls are falling apart, the floors are filthy and the lighting is terrible. The standard of cleanliness in their operating theatres is good but still far below what we expect in Canada. Their surgical team has just learned how to do laparoscopic procedures, and today a simple gall bladder removal took five times longer than it should have in well-trained hands. The interesting thing is that their surgeons don't seem to be interested in learning how to do these procedures more efficiently.

We also spent some time with the folks who will be organizing the children's party in Bihac where the Minister of National Defence will be giving out his shoeboxes. Operation Shoebox has become a buzzword that nearly everyone in the CAF has heard of. Given that the Minister is coming to help out, I have ceased calling Cpl Holland the "Shoebox Lady" and I am now referring to her as "Madame Shoebox." This evening a group of five of us helped to sort, categorize and wrap shoeboxes for the kids. We filled three Tri-Wall boxes, and that sure seemed like a lot of gifts to us. The airplanes are apparently bringing over fifty-seven more Tri-Walls, which will definitely be a handful. Hooah!

---

10 December 1998

Miracle of miracles! It has started to warm up a little and most of us are very happy about this change. I ordered some medical CDs a few weeks ago and they arrived today. One of them is called Interactive Skeleton and it allows you to take bones and joints and move them around in any direction you want. It should be a very useful learning tool provided I can find the time to use it regularly. At fourteen Deutsche Marks the price is impossible to beat.

The CO of the BG mentioned to me that the RSM had an electrocardiogram today and wanted to know what the results were. I was unaware of this having occurred, but since the RSM was standing right beside him, I decided to take advantage of the situation. I told the CO not to worry that the ECG registered absolutely no signal whatsoever, but that this confirms what the soldiers had been telling me all along. When he asked me what that might be, I replied, "That the RSM is a heartless old bastard." Fortunately, they both thought this was funny. Despite my teasing, the RSM is a great gentleman who exercises daily, and as such, leads by example.

Our intelligence people have learned of a new growth industry in Bosnia – it is called smuggling Kosovar refugees. Apparently the going rate to get into Croatia is 2-3,000 Deutsche Marks per Kosovar. It is amazing how one nation's disaster turns out to be a business opportunity for the unscrupulous.

There has been another soldier death in theatre, but this soldier was with the British contingent. It appears that he was standing between two armoured vehicles when they came together and accidentally crushed him. There will be at least one family in the world that won't be enjoying a Merry Christmas this year. I sincerely hope that we return home safely with the remainder of our troops.

This afternoon, an American Puma helicopter from Tuzla delivered a surgeon and a nurse anaesthetist to our camp. In exchange, we provided them with our general surgeon and Sleepy Doc who were flown back to visit the facilities in Tuzla. This is a great opportunity for both teams of personnel because they very rarely get to go anywhere, and when they do, it cannot be more than thirty minutes from the camp. I haven't seen Tuzla yet, but I am hoping to make this happen before I leave here.

---

11 December 1998

God smiled on Coralici this morning, and the temperatures have returned to something far more tolerable. While I was in the washroom this morning, one of the young captains came in, and after looking in the mirror declared, "I got rooster head!" A line like this was just too good to be true, so from my toilet stall I shouted out, "That's better than getting no head at all." That got his day off to a fine start. This was an RCR, and if you know any Regimental history, you'll know I could have had a great deal more fun with his statement than I did.

The aircraft designated to carry all the humanitarian aid are still scheduled to head over from Canada. In fact, the first flight is due to leave today. All together, they are expected to deliver somewhere between 55,000 and 60,000 pounds of aid for the contingent to distribute in the next seven weeks. I still cannot believe that this whole thing is really happening. It is especially rewarding to know that all the outstanding humanitarian aid is going to make it over because of Op Shoebox.

This evening, a military police officer arrived in camp and said, "You're the guy who's doing the humanitarian aid aren't you?" When I admitted my guilt, he told me that the international police unit in the town of Cazin have a room full of new toys and candy for children, and they were wondering if we would take them to distribute to kids in need. It's amazing how the spirit of giving just doesn't seem to want to stop. We will have to drop by and pick the stuff up, but I will likely have a hard time getting anyone to come with me because rumour has it that every time I drive anywhere, there is usually some kind of complication.

The situation in Kosovo continues to percolate, and through the winter months both sides will likely concentrate a great deal of effort on rearming themselves. Spring could be a very interesting time around here – I will be glad to be home before then. Against all advice, the American State Department decided to invest hundreds of millions of dollars to provide the Federation Army in Bosnia with modern weapons. Their objective was to try and restore the balance of power in the region and, in doing so, promote regional stability. Instead, they have equipped the Federation Army better than either the Serbs or the Croatians and have in fact managed to create even greater instability than before. Even the American army warned them this was a bad move, and now we will have to wait and see what will ultimately happen here. TGIF, and all that means is only two more working days until Monday.

---

12 December 1998

God has again blessed the "prisoners" of Stalag Coralici with outstanding weather.

We had to endure another lengthy BG meeting today during which the attendees dealt with every little detail of everything that is happening in the AOR. One thing for sure is that the BG knows about Op Shoebox and finally seems to be warming up to the project. From the discussion, it appears that handing the shoeboxes out to the children in Bihac will be one of the high points for the Minister of National Defence's visit, which has likely played more than a small role in the sudden warming of the 3 RCR to this non-operational distraction.

Given the fact that Bosnia remains a fairly dangerous place to work, Canadian soldiers are paid what is referred to as a hazard bonus. This contingent has had so many visits inflicted upon it that the standing joke is that the senior leadership is considering changing our hostility bonus to a hospitality bonus. Given the amount of work it takes catering to all these celebrities, we should get paid more for playing host than we do for dodging bullets and avoiding land mines.

Despite the unpredictable weather, our contingent continues to have to drive a great deal to perform its mission. To date our military vehicles have logged more than 1.6 million kilometres on the roads of Bosnia. To put that into perspective, that is an average of over 10,500 kilometres a day, which is a great deal of driving especially on the hazardous roads that are ubiquitous in this country.

I have come to understand that the Army spends so much time acting tough, when it comes time to be compassionate, some of its personnel appear to be incapable of being so. The other night a young soldier asked me if he could talk to me in my office. He then proceeded to tell me that his father was going to have coronary artery bypass surgery in five days' time. When I asked him how he felt about this, he burst into tears and told me that he was an only child and was terrified that his father would not survive the procedure. I took my time and explained that this is a very common procedure and that the cardiovascular surgeons have become so proficient at it that the risks are very small. This seemed to help him a great deal. He told me that he would never consider having a conversation like this with his superiors as they almost certainly would not understand and would likely criticize him for being so weak. It seems a little clearer to me why some combat soldiers choose to kill themselves rather than ask their chain of command for help.

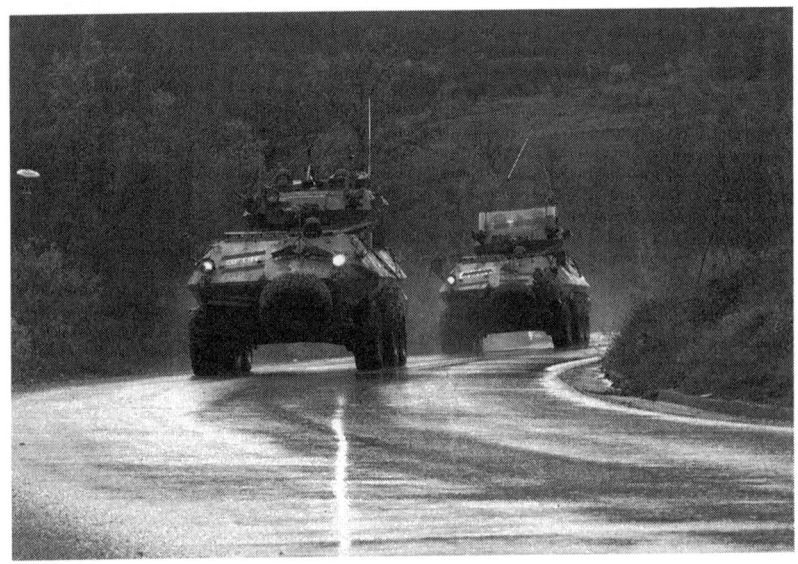

Canadian Forces soldiers spent an enormous amount of time on the roads of Bosnia and this driving was made dangerous by the weather conditions, the serpentine roads and reckless Bosnia drivers.

---

13 December 1998

'Twas another beautiful winter morning here in the badly damaged country of Bosnia, so some friends and I celebrated it by going for an eighty-two-minute run in the hills. We have developed a fairly loyal crew of running enthusiasts who can be counted on through the heat and cold. This is very nice because I would go crazy if I couldn't regularly get out of our camp and blow off some steam with exercise.

The monthly Commander's conference was held today, and I elected to put on a PowerPoint presentation to illustrate some of the health statistics for our tour thus far. In the process, I took a couple of cheap shots at the Army. The statistics show that Canadian soldiers see their medical staff 1.6 times more often than the average for other SFOR units. To explain this, I suggested there was likely a build-up of festering weakness in the troops. Oh, they loved hearing this from an Air Force puke. One of the Army personnel retorted with his own alternative explanation. He suggested that perhaps our medical staff were so incompetent that our patients had to see us more frequently to be cured. Touché! The Commander warned us that the last six weeks of our tour will be the most dangerous due to a combination of factors, which include personnel complacency and fatigue, in addition to the winter weather. He would like us all to remain focused and to carry the baton right to the finish line. I completely agree with him and will certainly try my best.

A team of us spent over two hours this evening packaging and wrapping shoeboxes. Cpl Holland is very well-organized, and people seem to just love working with her. She received a card tonight in which the sender thanked her for all her work and told her she was an angel – in my opinion they are absolutely right.

Stalag Coralici has its own amateur radio station that is manned by soldiers who volunteer to be DJs. This evening, the female DJ announced that "Jenny" had not been seen all day, and BG personnel are beginning to worry about her. This continued for quite a while before I finally asked one of the other people helping with the wrapping who Jenny was and what they thought was going on. She politely informed me that Jenny was a full-sized rubber woman that the ladies had purchased to accompany them wherever they went. Last night a young soldier was celebrating his birthday and the ladies lent him Jenny for the evening, and now they are wondering where the little tramp is hiding. I guess there is a whole other world going on in Stalag Coralici that this naïve and nearly prehistoric Air Force medical officer is completely unaware of.

---

14 December 1998

This evening we are being blessed with a light rain that appears to be forming a thin film of ice over everything. I can hardly wait to see what our morning run will have in store for all of the nutcases that are still pounding the pavement.

I had the opportunity to go up to the ambulanta in Todorovo this morning, and because of the weather, we only had five patients waiting to be seen. We saw a gentleman who was shot in the right side of his chest during the war and was now having trouble breathing. He has been told that he requires surgery because his right lung is adhered to its pleural lining. From the look of the exit wound on his back, he is lucky to be alive and able to walk. If the bullet had hit him an inch closer to the midline of his body, it would likely have shattered his spinal column. He told us that he was apprehensive about having the surgery done, and I sensed that he wanted some reassurance from me. I told him that it was obvious to me that God wanted him to survive his shooting, and so I am certain God will watch out for him during his surgery. I hope that this advice helped him make his decision.

We also saw a lady who was looking for formula for her one-month-old child. She told us that she was not breastfeeding the child because a witch had put a curse on her, and she was afraid that the curse could pass from her breast milk to her innocent young child. Our translator informed us that this is a very common way of thinking in the rural areas, and it was unlikely we would be able to convince the patient otherwise. As the interview went on, we discovered that in addition to being recently divorced, the mom was also on some psychiatric medications she did not want to share with her child via her breast milk. Ultimately, we gave her a large supply of infant formula, which is inferior to breast milk but a whole lot better than nothing at all.

As part of Op Shoebox, we brought gifts for each of the kids we saw. These were a big hit, and we will continue doing this while we are here.

This afternoon, I saw a very senior NCO (non-commissioned officer) who has been experiencing sciatica-like back pain for about a month, but despite our best efforts we have been unable to convince him that to get better he needs to slow down. The examination today showed that he cannot walk without a limp, and he has lost his left patellar reflex. While he was initially reluctant to be admitted, I explained to him that I was only making it sound like he had a choice in the matter – he got the picture. He will be with us for the next seven to ten days, and I hope the mandatory rest helps to relieve the pressure on his sciatic nerve otherwise he will likely be heading home.

---

15 December 1998

It's hard to believe that there are only ten days left until Christmas – Christmas without my nuclear family, mind you, but Christmas with my contingent family. Not quite the same thing, but better than nothing. The temperature this afternoon rose to what had to be plus 10°C and all the snow on the ground has melted into huge puddles. If it freezes tonight, we will have a multitude of small skating rinks all over the camp. Too bad we don't have any hockey equipment.

Things remain relatively quiet in the entire country of Bosnia. The intelligence boys informed us that an eighteen-year-old girl was killed this week when the grenade she was carrying in her pocket detonated. Old explosives can become unstable with time, and that is when tragedies like this can occur. I can't help asking myself why the hell a teenage girl would be walking around with a fully functional grenade in her pocket? Following this tragedy, her father turned in eight more grenades. It's too bad he hadn't decided to turn them in a few days earlier. I imagine this same thought will haunt this poor man for the rest of his life.

I spent a few hours this afternoon preparing cartons of shoeboxes for our medical teams to take to the ambulanta in Todorovo and the Bihac hospital. All our soldiers seem to be very excited about being able to give a Christmas gift to a Bosnian child. With Madame Shoebox away on R&R for the next four days, I guess that means I automatically become the "Shoebox Guy" – I just hope that the pressure of such responsibility doesn't overwhelm me.

In my wanderings around our camp, I have discovered that the maintenance platoon has adopted a puppy named "Stinky" who resides in their nice warm sprung shelter. This is strictly verboten at Stalag Coralici, but he is so darn cute that I can't imagine anyone giving him the boot. He sure looks a good deal healthier than the other abandoned dogs that wonder around the countryside desperately looking for something to eat.

Janet sounded lonely tonight, and I must admit that I am feeling the same way. I would like to spend more than fifteen minutes talking to the woman I love – about anything – without having to say, "Sorry, Honey, but we only have another thirty seconds." I shouldn't complain, considering that the personnel on our rotation have had more opportunities to communicate with family back home than any other rotation has ever had in Bosnia.

16 December 1998

Another relatively warm day in the war zone that the Bosnian people call home. This morning the road was covered with a very thin layer of ice, and although we cautioned them to do their workout on the road, the RSM and camp commandant elected to go for a run in the hills. Apparently, they nearly killed themselves. Upon their return, they declared that until further notice, personnel will only be permitted to run off the camp between 0900 and 1600hrs. It amazes me that their misadventure has translated into depriving the other early morning runners from the opportunity to sneak in a good workout while the rest of the camp personnel get some much-needed beauty sleep. I know their intention was well meant but this decree will certainly make life more difficult for those of us who use our early morning runs to preserve what little mental health we still have left.

It would appear that Bosnia and Croatia are having a dispute over borderlines in our AOR, and the Croatian police have been pointing their long-barreled weapons at our troops. As part of a well-orchestrated disinformation campaign, the Croatian media is broadcasting how Canadian soldiers are trying to ignite trouble by pointing their weapons at the Croatian police. This is very frustrating for us all especially because Croatia is making less-than-subtle efforts to try and grab large portions of Bosnia. If this continues, there will likely be significant troubles in contested regions of the country, and Canadian soldiers will likely have to become involved. If this does happen, I sure hope none of our boys get hurt.

This afternoon, our staff had the distinct pleasure of excising shrapnel from a soldier's buttocks. Apparently, as a young boy he was playing with a twenty-two round, and when it exploded, pieces of it were embedded in various parts of his body. He wanted this particular piece removed because it was starting to hurt when he was sitting. For your average soldier, sitting is a surprisingly large part of the day.

Sgt Buchanan is our 6A medical assistant (senior medical assistant), and he did the entire procedure while I simply looked over his shoulder. I spent a year doing experimental surgery and I could not have done a better job.

The Battle Group has just published the formal instructions for the distribution of the Christmas shoeboxes, and while I am one of the co-directors for this project, my name does not appear in either the document or the distribution list. I would like to believe that this was an accidental oversight, but I think this omission is reflective of the Army's displeasure at having an outsider involved in this entire project. Even if that outsider helped play a major role in getting them involved in this wonderful project. Give me the Air Force any day.

---

17 December 1998

This morning I had the mind-numbing pleasure of repeatedly running three-minute circles around the inside of our camp as a result of the decision that the CO of the BG made yesterday. I am surprised that I wasn't dizzy by the end of the workout. The tragedy is that I was, in fact, the only person out running, and when I went to the gymnasium, the only other person there was also from the medical staff. As it turns out, the only people who had been in the gymnasium prior to 0800hrs were support staff – cooks and medics. It appears that not a single person from the Army managed to haul their rear ends out of bed to exercise this morning. It is possible that they all worked very late and needed the extra rack time this morning. Perhaps they are all planning to do their workouts later in the day when the gym and the running trails aren't quite so crowded. Or perhaps weakness is starting to invade our camp and the first symptom we are seeing is a drop in morning PT.

This afternoon I received my big CANEX Christmas gift box, which every deployed Canadian soldier is supposed to receive. It is a nice idea. The box contains candies, a track bag, a ball cap and all kinds of other goodies. This will be another gift I can put under my own Christmas tree – if I ever find the time to make one.

The bombing of Iraq was the big news today. No one seems to feel that it will have much of an impact on the level of threat directed at SFOR soldiers. I am not as certain of this, given the fact that one of the local Muslim medical clinics is named after Saddam himself.

The border conflict between Bosnia and Croatia continues, and I think it is likely to continue as long as there is at least one Bosnian and one Croatian on the face of the earth. If these disputes heat up, I hope that none of our troops get injured in the fracas.

I have spent most of the afternoon and all evening preparing thank-you letters for all the folks who made significant contributions to my medical supplies project. This was tiring, but I am glad it is finally completed. I am pooped, so I think I will go and press my face deeply into my pillow while the overworked Army guys play games in the Mess.

---

18 December 1998

It has been a busy and exciting day for little old me. It started off with yet another lonely jog in the fog. Then, after our weekly Commander's briefing in Camp Maple Leaf (VK) I was informed that the medical team had found my humanitarian medical supplies and had stored them adjacent to the gymnasium. It was very exciting to see seven and a half Tri-Walls of stuff that we had fought so hard to get to Bosnia, sitting right in front of me. A group of us emptied every Tri-Wall and then sorted out the items to be given to the Todorovo clinic, the pediatric clinic in Velika Kladusa, and the Velika Kladusa and Bihac hospitals. It was wonderful to see all the practical supplies that were there. I am particularly looking forward to giving all these supplies to the pediatrician who thought that I was one of those people who promises lots and delivers nothing. Hopefully what we provide her with will allow her to better treat her patients for more than one year. It was nice to see that our medical assistants also seemed to be excited about the arrival of our much-needed medical supplies. On the downside, it appears that only half of Cpl Holland's shoeboxes have been flown into theatre, and there are still another thirty Tri-Walls that will hopefully be loaded on to a plane headed this way tomorrow. My experience to date has made me somewhat of a doubting Thomas even though I know the Lord would like me to trust Him more on this.

Cpl Holland and I were both interviewed by the Ottawa Valley media currently touring the AOR. Mike McHugh, a reporter who lives in Russell, also interviewed me. It was nice to hear his voice and get a chance to let everyone at home know that the humanitarian aid program is going very well. It was also a chance to wish everyone back home a Merry Christmas.

The Minister of Defence and the Colonel-in-Chief of the RCR both arrived in our camp this evening because their helicopters could not land in VK. This was unanticipated and I am sure this sudden change of plans caused a whole lot of people a whole lot of work.

Another big day scheduled for tomorrow, so I had better get some sleep to reduce the chances of me falling asleep while playing the role of Santa Claus.

---

19 December 1998

It truly has been a big day, and I was already exhausted before it had even started. The weather here has been unbelievably nice for the last few days, and I would guess that the high today must have reached 12°C. I was mentioning to one of our Newfoundland medical assistants that my daughter Rebecca would like to become an artist. He looked at me with a straight face and replied, "All of my relatives are artists – they're all drawing unemployment." Ouch! In a similar vein, someone gave me a card today that says, "You know that you have been really bad when" and when you open it up, it shows Santa sitting down for a crap on your chimney. It appears that this is the time of year when everyone is out to "slag" their fellow man – an approach which is consistent with the charitable Christmas ideal of "It is better to give than to receive."

We had the big Christmas party in Bihac today, and it was a very well-organized event. The Op Shoebox team under the supervision of Corporal Holland (alias Colonel Holland) is truly well prepared. The event was held in a small sports centre and was sandwiched between physical spaces being used for a Ping-Pong tournament. A team of about twenty-five of us went down by bus with four Tri-Walls containing approximately four hundred shoeboxes. We needed an hour to set up, and then the doors were opened. It was obvious before we even began setting up that we may have underestimated the popularity of the event, as

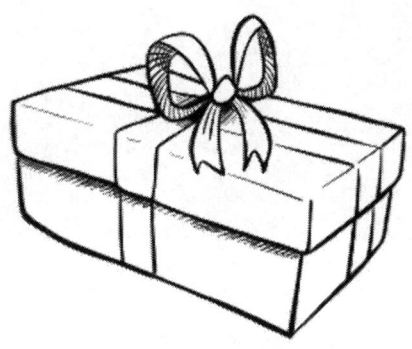

A typical Christmas shoebox

people were already lining up. We decided to send a vehicle back to pick up more shoeboxes, which turned out to be a very good idea because otherwise we would have run out of gifts before we ran out of children.

I was asked to come out dressed as Santa about fifteen minutes before the Minister of National Defence was scheduled to arrive. I am not a very big person so I looked less like jolly old St. Nick and more like Scrawny old Santa. When I made my entrance, the crowd immediately surrounded me. Everyone wanted me to touch their child. I patted as many on the head as I could and wished them all a Merry Christmas. After plowing my way through the pressing throng, I finally made it to Santa's chair in front of the mountainous pile of presents. The idea was to have each child sit on my knee and pose for an instant Polaroid

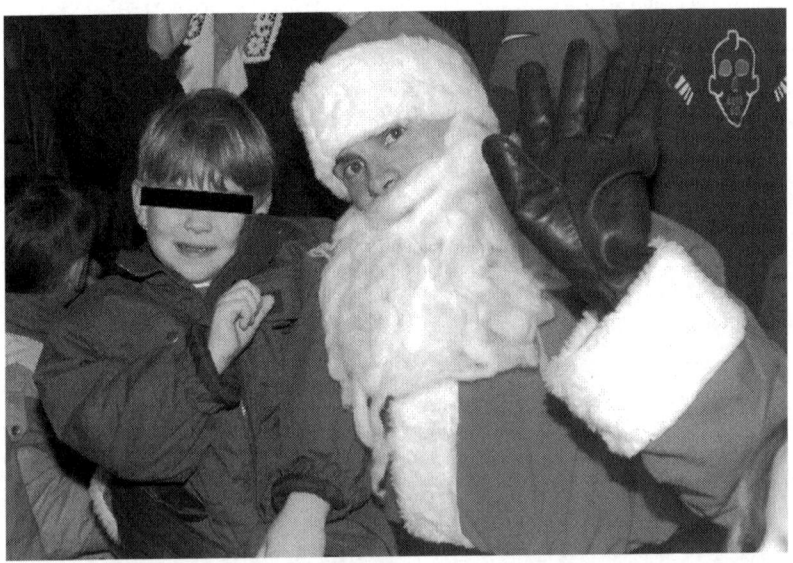

Me dressed in the Santa Claus suit my wife sent from Canada. This was one of the many Christmas parties set up by Cpl Holland and her team of volunteers.

picture while receiving their gifts. This was difficult because the crowd completely surrounded me, and everyone wanted their child to be held next. Our soldiers literally had to employ crowd control measures to ensure that Santa and his helpers weren't completely overrun. It was wild. About fifteen minutes into my routine, the Minister arrived at my side and said, "Don't stop what you are doing, this is a day for the children." I grabbed him and had him sit on my knee with a bunch of children, and the photographers went to town. I didn't see him again, but apparently, he spent ten minutes talking to Cpl Holland about her project before continuing on his merry way along with his entourage of security personnel. When all was said and done, everyone was stunned by the popularity of the event, not to mention completely drained. Thank you, Lord, for helping us to make this a very special day for so many children.

---

20 December 1998

I got up early today to head off to VK with a work party to break down the twenty-two Tri-Walls of shoeboxes in storage there. We need these shoeboxes to be given as gifts for two children's parties that will be held tomorrow in Drvar. The work party was enthusiastic, and it only took us two hours to sort everything out. Unfortunately, only about half of the Tri-Walls contained unwrapped shoeboxes or supplies that could be used to make up shoeboxes. This was disappointing, but we kept our fingers crossed that the plane that landed this morning in Zagreb would have the remaining three thousand shoeboxes. We waited around for four hours only to discover that there wasn't a single shoebox on the flight that had landed. What the cargo did contain was the remaining six Tri-Walls of my medical supplies and all the clothing boxes from the great town of Russell. It was impossible for me to celebrate the final delivery of my stuff when Corporal Holland had been let down so badly. The saddest part of all this is that my stack of supplies and clothing could have waited till next week – if someone had prioritized these items, we might have seen all the much-needed shoeboxes arrive on time.

There is a Hercules aircraft flying here tomorrow, and we are told that it will be carrying the remainder of the humanitarian aid that was still sitting in Trenton. If this is true, then it should literally be an entire load of shoeboxes. We couldn't call to change things around even if we wanted to because the load has already been prepared and wrapped. We will have to leave it in God's hands and wait until tomorrow night to find out what materials made it over the pond. In an effort to adapt to the uncertain situation we find ourselves in, the parties in Drvar have been delayed for two days. If the shoeboxes are not on tomorrow's flight, we will have to change numerous plans because there are no more flights scheduled for this theatre until the 28th of December, and that flight will likely be full of items needed by our operators to fix or maintain their big boy toys.

There was a huge quantity of mail delivered today, and I got four packages of blessings from friends and loved ones. I look forward to opening them up in five days, but it will not be the same without Janet, the kids and the cats. Hooah!

---

21 December 1998

The shortest day of the year has come and gone, and we will finally start to see the sun rising earlier and earlier. The road conditions had improved to the point that we were finally going to be allowed to run off the base again. This all went to hell in a handbasket when Mother Nature dumped another huge volume of snow on us. It snowed so much that the all-weather Sea King helicopter out of Sipovo could not pick up three patients we wanted to have assessed in Rajlovac. So this morning, I wasted one hour of my life sitting on the frozen helicopter landing zone waiting for nothing.

The roads were very treacherous, and consequently, there were countless cars in ditches and numerous accidents. One of those accidents involved a civilian vehicle hitting one of our huge HLVW (Heavy Logistic Vehicle Wheeled) trucks – essentially ten tons of metal. One of the occupants of the car died in one of our soldier's arms, and the other is reported to be in critical condition. Apparently, the civilians were driving way too fast for the road conditions and lost control of the vehicle as they attempted to pass the HLVW. Their car was demolished, but the HLVW was hardly scratched.

Today was the RCR's birthday and they celebrated it as only the Army can – with a parade at 0900hrs in the middle of a snowstorm. True to the Army's obsessive-compulsive nature, the soldiers were all lining up for the event one hour before anything happened. To rub salt into the wounds, the soldiers were ordered to take off their gloves and stand for one hour in the freezing cold. This unpleasant order was given so that the soldiers could shake hands with the Colonel of the Regiment who would be presenting each of them with their tour medal. If this is called putting your soldiers first, I would hate to see what second place looks like.

We had a surprise visitor in the UMS this morning. Apparently, Jenny the rubber doll had finally returned from her trip to Bootie-Fest and the little scamp was sporting a brand-new tattoo. The ladies accompanying her ensured she was in full uniform and wanted me to give her a physical to confirm that she hadn't caught anything "nasty" on her excursion with the boys. I gave her a thorough looking over and pronounced her "fit to philander" once again.

I have learned to weave using paracord (parachute cord) so I have started putting knotted pieces of rope onto everything that I own. This is guaranteed to get under the skin of the army hard-liners. I love it.

I spent the evening making shoeboxes and wrapping them. We still haven't heard if the remaining boxes were flown into Zagreb this evening. I sure hope that they were, or it will be a real blow to Corporal Holland and all her supporters. The National Post did a telephone interview with me this evening and wanted to know the entire medical aid story. I hope that the CF gets a little positive PR from all this.

Good night my loved ones on the other side of the world.

Here is a little Christmas poem I composed. I think it is very appropriate for this time of year and would like to share with the folks back at home. I believe it reflects how many military personnel who are isolated from our loved ones feel at this time of year.

"My Gift is My Service"

It's hard to believe that it's Christmas Day
And I am deployed in a land quite far away.
My home is a sea container that's been modified
It's cold in the winter and in the summer I fried.

No presents, no tree, no holiday lights
No loved ones, in the kitchen cooking Yuletide delights.
As a Canadian peacekeeper I don't expect more
There's a price to be paid protecting others from war.

It's been a long tour and I miss being home.
Time seems to move slower when you live alone.
Christmas should be enjoyed with family and friends
Not spent in a tin can praying war would soon end.

What I wouldn't give for a hug and a kiss
And a chance to spend time with the loved ones I miss.

But my family will have to celebrate on their own
The best I can do is to call on the phone.

God, please keep my family safe while I am away
Help them know I think of them every day.
Your son died on a cross that we all might live
I can't think of a greater gift anyone could give.

Christmas is another workday for this tired soldier
Protecting innocent people from a life of disorder.
With no presents to send home, my love will have to do.
My gift is my service – that's my gift to you!

Merry Christmas everyone

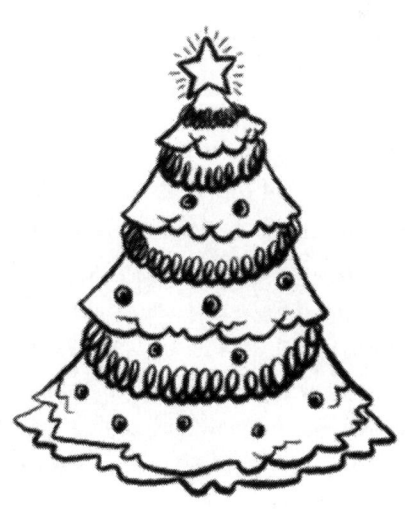

22 December 1998

It has been a very busy day here in Stalag Coralici, and I am really very tired. It is difficult to find the energy to do everything that needs to be done. I have discovered that the boys in the UMS have started to refer to us as "trailer trash" because we live in sea containers. You know you have hit rock bottom when people start calling you trailer trash and it doesn't bother you.

This afternoon the helicopter boys finally managed to take off to transport two of our patients to the German hospital for their CT scans. I suspect that they each have a disc herniation, which will not be great news for either of them. This evening, we were informed that our patients are stranded in Sarajevo because our helicopter was tasked away for an urgent operational requirement. Logistic problems like this are no one's fault but they do make providing good medical care in theatre a constant challenge.

In the afternoon, I travelled up to our camp in VK to ensure that all our medical donations were appropriately divided up and distributed. Ultimately, we collected sixteen Tri-Walls of useful supplies. Tomorrow at 1530hrs, the Commander and I will deliver the supplies to the VK hospital. I sincerely hope that the local medical staff there appreciate all the effort that has gone into this undertaking. We will deliver the remaining supplies to the hospital in Bihac on the following day. While in VK, I also stopped by to help the troops who were breaking down the thirty-five Tri-Walls of shoeboxes that, thankfully, were delivered the day before. These boxes were not as well-organized as we had been led to believe, so the team had to do a great deal of sorting. In the end, we were lacking about 150 presents for the older children who would be receiving shoeboxes tomorrow. This left only one option – our team spent three hours in the evening putting together, from scratch, the 150 boxes that were needed. While this would normally be an enjoyable activity, I could see that everyone involved was tired before we had even begun. Bless them all, because not one person said they were getting worn out.

Tonight, I was informed that a British Lynx helicopter had crashed, and three crew members were injured. This is the third helicopter that has gone down since we have been here – it sure makes you appreciate how dangerous flying in this mountainous region is. I hope that these soldiers completely recover from their injuries.

A very large percentage of soldiers are taking the opportunity to get tattooed while in theatre. While the prices appear to be excellent, in my opinion the craftmanship is mediocre at best. The soldiers are all coming into the UMS and asking for Polysporin to lather onto these masterpieces. Hooah! Hooah!

The entire contingent is winding up for a very dangerous operation that will be launched in the early morning hours. They fully anticipate that there could be casualties, so our alert status will increase substantially. This has turned our Christmas season into a time of worry instead of a time of peace. Our media people informed Corporal Holland and me that the National Post reporter was very impressed with the humanitarian work being done by the Canadian Contingent. He said that he was very proud of our soldiers, and that is something we sure don't hear very often from the Canadian media.

---

23 December 1998

The flags in our camp are once again flying at half-mast. It appears that after the British helicopter went down, two of the crew members eventually died, and one remains in critical condition. This brings the British soldier death toll to six in the last six months and the total number of deaths in our Division to eleven. That is a staggering average of one death every two weeks. The

Battle Group's secret mission is now complete, so I can talk about it. In the Martin Brod region, the Croatians have been illegally occupying a portion of Bosnia, and their police have been patrolling it. SFOR tasked the 3 RCR Battle Group with going in and removing the Croatian security element using whatever force was required. This type of confrontation in a highly volatile region had the real potential for gunfire and casualties. The Battle Group wanted the element of surprise on their side, and so the security for this operation was quite strict. We know that the Croatian Forces have intelligence sources in all of our camps. H-hour (the time set for the beginning of a planned attack) was 0400hrs this morning, and employing the tactical elements of surprise and overwhelming numbers, the Battle Group achieved its mission without any gunfire. The Croatian security forces peacefully complied with their eviction, and since they had no vehicles, our lads actually had to give them a lift to the real borderline before letting them out to walk home. This is a great victory and certainly a big relief to everyone, as we sure didn't want to be dealing with World War III at Christmas time. Merci, Lord.

We delivered eight Tri-Walls of medical supplies to the VK hospital this afternoon, and the staff there seemed very appreciative of the generous donation from the people of Russell. They were especially grateful to receive all very practical materials. All too often they get junk that no one else wants or items that are stale-dated. The Commander came for the photo opportunity and the hospital director told us how important Canadian soldiers were to the peace process here in Bosnia. As our Commander put it, Christmas is the time for giving, and our soldiers have chosen to give the people of Bosnia peace – I hope that Canadians remember the enormous price tag that some of our colleagues paid in order to provide this generous gift.

24 December 1998

Tis the night before Christmas, and I got to enjoy one of the busiest clinical days I have had since we first came into theatre. I also had the eight Tri-Walls of medical supplies delivered to the Bihac hospital, whose staff seemed very grateful for the donations. I ended up running all over the place until 1600hrs, and the ASC's Christmas gift exchange was scheduled to begin at 1630hrs. To complicate matters, I had not yet got my gag gift ready and wrapped, and I still had to jump into my Santa suit. Through some miracle of time suspension, I actually made it with time to spare. The gift exchange was a real hoot for everyone who was there. People were supposed to buy a gift for twenty dollars or less and place it under the ASC Christmas tree. At the exchange you could then elect to pick a gift from under the tree or steal one from someone who had already opened a gift. If your gift was stolen, you were free to steal someone else's gift. You can imagine all the backstabbing that went on. As Santa Claus, my role was to be the conductor of this three-ring circus.

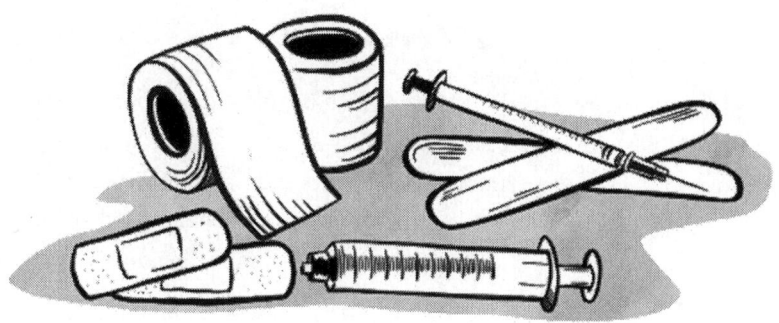

Medical supplies from Russell Ontario

Following the gift exchange, I got into my uniform and helped set up the chapel for midnight Mass. This service was an even bigger deal than usual because the Chief of the Defence Staff (CDS) was in attendance. After that we had a choir practice and then walked all over the camp caroling to the soldiers who were still on duty. We then went to the mess to meet the CDS who arrived over an hour later than anticipated. While he seems to be motivated to spend time with his troops, he certainly cannot be described as a very colourful or inspiring individual. I didn't have the opportunity to say a word to him, let alone make any eye contact, and I can't tell you how much that broke my heart. Not!

From that exciting moment in my life, we moved back to the chapel where, as part of the choir, I had the opportunity to participate in one of the nicest midnight Mass celebrations I have ever seen. There was such a radiant atmosphere in the room. Part of my tiny brain must be turning combat green because I really didn't notice how odd it was to be celebrating Mass with everyone in uniform. It sure would be nice to be able to go home for just one night.

---

25 December 1998

Merry Christmas to all. I started the day off right by phoning Janet and the kids at 0115hrs their time. This was quite a surprise since I fully expected to spend most of the day dialing the phone in an effort to reach my precious loved ones. They all sound to be in good spirits, and I hope that they are enjoying themselves rather than sitting around wishing I were there with them.

As is my custom, I got up this morning and went for a run in the hills with my buds. It was great to get off the camp and enjoy this special day that the Lord has given to humankind.

I spent most of the day putzing around the camp wishing everyone a Merry Christmas. This afternoon we celebrated with a very old military tradition whereby the officers and senior NCOs serve Christmas dinner to the troops. As part of this evening, a unit often sings carols to the dining troops. This year, members of the ASC staff spent a great deal of time coming up with new lyrics for old songs. I was given the chance to review them prior to the dinner, and while there were a few lines that I think transcended the bounds of good taste, the majority of the musical entertainment was very funny. Unfortunately, not everyone thought the songs were appropriate, so then the medical staff were not allowed to sing anything. As you can imagine, this made for some very disappointed health care providers.

While the dinner went well, several of us were left with the distinct impression that this event was a mere formality, and there was very little sincerity behind it. It was just another formal distraction designed to break Christmas Day into an unending chain of formal obligations rather than a period of relaxation for everyone. I have simply refused to get excited over any of the pomp and circumstance that other well-intentioned people have spent their entire day worrying about. Despite my pessimistic attitude, I sincerely hope this event helped reduce the heartache of spending Christmas away from home for some of our soldiers.

Sitting here, I realize just how very tired I am. I am very much looking forward to a few days off in Bled, Slovenia, even to just sleep in, take a hot bath, read more and maybe try to cross-country ski. No matter how I slice it, today is just not the same without Janet, Nath, Kim, Matt, Jenny, Becky, BB, Baby and Skye.

Happy Birthday, Lord, and thank you for coming into the world so that we may have the opportunity to enjoy eternal life with you.

26 December 1998

Boxing Day in theatre is like any other holiday – you have work to do and people to take care of. Christmas night, more of our soldiers deployed to the Martin Brod region – I have been here so long now that it took me awhile to realize how abnormal this actually is. I am sure this was not the kind of Christmas Day most of these soldiers had envisioned. I guess we all need to remember that we are working in a very, very unusual place and that's all there is to it.

This was the big day when those who will be leaving first had to deliver their unaccompanied baggage to be loaded into sea containers. All such material will be sent to Canada ahead of the departing soldiers. This activity is yet another reminder that our time here in Bosnia is rapidly coming to a close. I will be one of the very last to leave – it will be hard to see my friends go and then have to break in a group of rookies.

We had our last series of Christmas parties for Bosnian children today, and these events were once again very well received. Parties were held in VK, Zgon and Cazin, and probably two thousand shoeboxes were hand-delivered to children by Canadian soldiers. I assisted at the event in Cazin where we were told that 130 children would be in attendance. In the end, we gave out nearly four hundred gifts and put a smile on a whole bunch of faces, both young and old. It is moments like these that clearly show how Canadians truly are worldwide ambassadors of peace, and it sure makes you proud to be a part of it. This really was the wrap-up day for Operation Shoebox, and those of us who have been heavily committed can all take a much-needed break.

The completion of Operation Shoebox could not have come at a better time for me because this evening I am leaving for ninety-six hours of R&R in Bled, Slovenia. Everyone tells me that there is nothing to do in Bled and that I will be bored out of my mind. This would be a remarkable feat, as I am quite certain that I am already out of my mind. At this point in my deployment, having nothing to do for ninety-six hours sounds pretty darn good to me. It is with considerable embarrassment that I confess that I will not be going to Bled alone. The ladies told me that Jenny the inflatable rubber lady wanted me to personally show her a wild time in Slovenia. I have also had to promise to bring her back with a new tattoo. This should be fun. They have actually given her a last name – she will henceforth be formally known as "Jenny Tuls." What a bunch of degenerates I am forced to work with. It seems hypocritical to call other people degenerates when you're the one travelling to Slovenia with a rubber woman in your suitcase. I sure as hell hope that my luggage doesn't get searched at the border. Can you imagine the scandalous news headlines that would create?

---

27 December 1998

A busload of us left Coralici for our R&R last night at about 2200hrs. We arrived in VK only to be told to form up in three ranks and "Relax!" In this natural state of relaxation, we were given a pre-departure briefing that basically stated we would be getting up at 0200hrs so that we could be given a departure briefing prior to getting on to a bus at 0300hrs. I believe the Army's secret intention here is to be certain that all of us are totally wiped out before we head off to be rejuvenated. Unlike many of the others, I managed to sneak in a refreshing two and a half hours of blissful sleep on the floor of the MIR.

At 0300hrs, the bright-eyed and bushy-tailed bunch of us were informed that the large and comfortable-looking tour bus we were supposed to be on had broken down, and our departure would be delayed by forty-five minutes. When that time was up, we were told that the bus could not be repaired, and we would have to travel in a military bus. We all loaded our luggage onto the bus and tried to find a comfortable place in the frozen green beast we were going to spend the next three hours bouncing around in. As we went to leave, we were unable to budge because the brake system on the bus had frozen. Plan C then kicked into gear, so we off-loaded all our stuff and climbed into an alternate frozen green beast. You can imagine our surprise when we discovered that this bus was actually capable of moving both forward and backward. What we didn't know until we were halfway to Zagreb was that the heating system wasn't working. Everyone was approaching a state of hypothermia when we finally arrived in Zagreb at 0600hrs. From there, six of us were jammed into a minivan and driven to Bled. This vehicle was also blessed with a dysfunctional heater, and by the time we arrived at our hotel, every last one of us was dog-tired and chilled to the bone. Maybe the real purpose of this exercise is to somehow make Stalag Coralici appear more attractive to those of us who are sentenced there.

After a mercifully short check-in, I ran upstairs and drew a boiling hot bath into which I immersed myself for half an hour. I then collapsed into a very comfortable bed and slept until noon. When I finally awoke, I had a whole new perspective on life. The weather had warmed considerably, and I went for a gorgeous run around the lake the town of Bled is built beside. Bled is located in the Julian Alps, and the scenery is absolutely breathtaking. Running at altitude is also a breathtaking experience.

It was immediately apparent that the community atmosphere in Bled is completely different from that of Bosnia. The area is affluent, the people are friendly and the facilities cater to a tourist clientele. I even got to watch part of a hockey practice, and I realized how much I enjoyed working with my kids' hockey teams all those years. I ate dinner at a nice Chinese restaurant and then enjoyed an evening of lying in bed and watching some mindless television. It sure would have been nice to share the evening with Janet. Please Lord, watch over everyone back home.

28 December 1998

Another beautiful day here in the Julian Alps. I had the entire day to myself, and it was nice just to flit around and accomplish very little. It's funny that you never know how tired you really are until you go somewhere to relax for a few days, and you end up crashing. It's obvious to me that my batteries were overdue for a recharge.

In the afternoon, I went for a two-hour walk in the forest and it was an absolutely awesome adventure. The smell of pine trees in the air, the crunching of snow underfoot, the brilliance of the sun and the supreme peace and quiet were all good for my weary soul. As I wandered along, I happened to scare a white-tailed deer and had the privilege of watching this graceful creature effortlessly leap through the woods to put as much distance between the two of us as possible. As an athlete, I have always found moments like this humbling because I know that I could train all my life and never achieve the physical perfection that I had just witnessed. In the evening, I went to a hockey game between the Bled club and a team from somewhere in Italy. The Italian team had a whole bunch of lads whose last names ended in "o" or "i". They also had two guys named Reid and Campbell. Figuring these might be Canadian lads, I went down to the bench between the first and second periods. It turns out that I was right – Reid is from Sault Ste. Marie and Campbell is from Kitchener. It was an entertaining game, but the Italian squad lost in overtime because Reid got lazy and let go of his check. It's good to see that Canadian boys still play Canadian-style hockey in Europe. The rest of my lazy evening was spent lying in bed watching a Discovery Channel special on our friend the shark. Think of all the fun I am missing in Bootie-Fest!

---

29 December 1998

Only one more month before my replacement arrives in theatre. It was another absolutely beautiful day here in Bled. The sun was out, the temperature was mild, and there was virtually no wind. I slept in until 0830hrs and awoke to find myself beginning to develop the symptoms of a cold. This had started a week ago in Coralici, but after my daily morning run, the symptoms would simply disappear. It is almost as though my body was saying, "You don't have time to be sick right now" and has been holding things off. Letting myself relax here seems to have allowed weakness to overwhelm my immune system, and now I will be paying the price for the next week or so. Once I finished blowing my nose, I went downstairs for a leisurely breakfast.

In the afternoon I had a great run around the lake and through part of the forest. Everywhere you go, there are people of every age out enjoying a walk around the lake. They seem to celebrate Christmas at a different time of year from Canadians, and interestingly, Santa was scheduled to make his grand entrance today. We knew that something was up because there have been church bells, music and firecrackers going off all day long. Now that I am just starting to enjoy this drastic change in lifestyle, I will be forced to head back to Stalag Coralici tomorrow morning. It hardly seems fair, but I must remain focused on the mission for a little while longer.

I took Jenny out of the bag this evening and gave her a stylized Bled tattoo just above her left breast. I think the ladies are going to pass Ms. Jenny Tuls on from one rotation to the next in the hopes that she will eventually have tattoos all over.

Lord, I am not looking forward to the trip back to Bosnia tomorrow, but I must admit it will be interesting to hear about all the things that happened while I was away.

30 December 1998

I am writing this note from the safety of my office in Coralici, but getting back home was once again quite the adventure. We were scheduled to head home at 0830hrs and so I got up at 0615hrs to say goodbye to beautiful Bled in the best way I know – with a solitary run. While I was eating breakfast, I was informed we would be leaving an hour later than planned. I was joined for breakfast by three of the most hungover rats you have ever seen. These young soldiers apparently finished partying around 0500hrs, and one of them had no idea where his socks or underwear were. This was apparently the first time they had seen the light of day since we arrived in Bled.

When our vehicle finally arrived, it turned out to be a five-passenger van, but there were seven of us to transport. We all crammed into this mobile sardine can, and the alcohol fumes were so heavy that had I lit a match, we probably would have gone up in smoke. Since we were somewhat behind schedule, our driver decided to try and make up time by driving at 195 kilometres an hour. When we asked him to slow down, he reluctantly decelerated to 160 kilometres an hour and continued weaving his way through the fast-moving traffic. We had one pit stop, but we couldn't buy anything because we had spent all of our tolars (Slovenian currency) and no other currency was accepted.

Our rendezvous with the tour bus was one hour later than scheduled because our driver had no idea where he was going in Zagreb. When we got on the bus, the temperature was approaching plus 40°C. When we asked the driver to turn the heat off, he thought we said "up" and soldiers began to experience "melt down." To add insult to injury, the bus showed the worst movie I had ever seen in my entire life. I am sure the production company saved a great deal of money by having no plot and no real actors for the film. I was the only one in our group who had brought a lunch because I had anticipated problems and didn't want to go hungry all day long. Why do these kind of travel problems always seem to happen to me? I must say that Stalag Coralici is a slum compared to Bled, and I sure am glad that my sentence is nearly up.

Corporal Holland's efforts on Operation Shoebox were honoured today when she was presented with a Contingent Commander's Commendation. Well deserved, Kim!

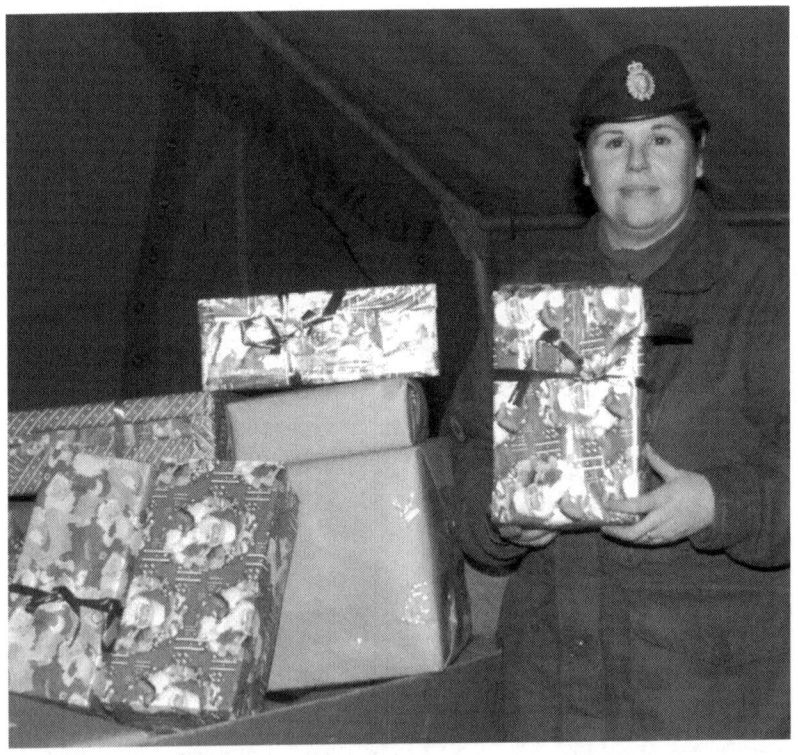

Cpl Kim Holland holding one of the thousands of Christmas shoeboxes that were delivered to Bosnian children as a result of her inspiration, motivation and hard work. She is truly a remarkable person.

31 December 1998

New Year's Eve, and I have no desire to be out celebrating the coming of 1999. I don't feel depressed in any way, I would just rather be spending this day with my family. My first New Year's Eve task was to return Jenny to her guardians, and I reassured them Jenny was returning to them with her virtuous reputation intact. From the looks on their faces, I am not convinced they believed me.

Our intelligence briefing this evening informed us that the situation in Kosovo is becoming increasingly violent once again, and I imagine before long the situation will be right back to square one. The resumption of fighting here will help absolutely no one.

This morning one of our large fuel trucks carrying approximately nine thousand litres of fuel went off the road and fell 150 metres before being stopped by trees. Somehow, the vehicle crew managed to jump ship before the vehicle fell. As if this wasn't miraculous enough, the truck didn't explode despite landing in a minefield with the motor still running and thousands of litres of fuel spilled all over hell's half acre. These were two extraordinarily lucky people, and I only hope they stop to thank God for taking care of them.

I elected to go to New Year's Mass this evening, and the two of us in the congregation were able to enjoy an intimate celebration the likes of which few people ever get a chance to experience.

My cold seems to be getting the better of me, and I am certain that it's all because of the hot baths that I enjoyed while I was in Bled. It must have given weakness the opportunity to soak in through my open pores and establish itself in my battle-hardened body. I am hoping that a few days in Stalag Coralici will demoralize the virus to the point that it willingly leaves my body.

We have begun doing the redeployment medicals for everyone in theatre, which should keep us busy for a few weeks. These medicals are called post-deployment medicals, and as such, should be done when we land on Canadian soil. The reality is that we are so short of medical staff, the majority of the work needs to be done in theatre, or else the receiving units would be literally overwhelmed. This situation is certain to get much worse before it gets better because given that our government leaders seem to be more reactive than they are proactive.

January 1999

1 January 1999

The flags in our camp are once again flying at half-mast because the third soldier who was injured in the recent crash of the British helicopter died last night. This sure has been a tough tour in terms of soldier fatalities.

My New Year's Eve night was rather interesting in that sometime between midnight and 0200hrs the power cord to my sea container and two others shorted out. At about 0200hrs I was awakened by a strange sound, and as I came to consciousness, I realized that what I was hearing was the chattering of my teeth. It was extremely cold in the tin can I call home and I still had to survive four more hours before my early morning run. I put on my fleece clothing and crawled under my covers and shivered vigorously until my alarm finally went off.

Getting dressed in near-total darkness on an ice-cold floor certainly does nothing to improve one's quality of life here in beautiful Stalag Coralici. It wasn't until I stepped outside that I was able to verify that I was wearing the correct clothing and that I hadn't put it on inside out or backwards. When I finished my workout, I was rewarded with a cold shower and the opportunity to dry off and dress in my refrigerated sea container. This would have been considerably more miserable if the weather outside had been really cold. I must admit that this is not what the doctor ordered to help me recover from my flu-like illness. I will likely be on my deathbed by tomorrow morning. On the other hand, it is also possible that the virus causing my illness froze to death last night and I will experience a miraculous recovery.

The repair crew managed to fix the wiring this evening, and my room is once again too hot. I won't complain because being overly warm beats being overly cold when you are living in an uninsulated tin can in the middle of winter.

I am certain that the CDS (Chief of Defence Staff) intended his Christmas visit to Bosnia to be a demonstration of support to the troops who are deployed away from home during this special time of the year. While this was a noble gesture, his presence in our camp turned our relaxation time into one huge hosting obligation. To reflect their true appreciation for his electing to spend his Christmas with us, some of the troops have decided CDS really means "Christmas Day spoiled." It is too bad that no one in the entire organization, including me, has the *cojones* to tell him the truth about this issue.

Despite the above, I had the rare opportunity to talk to Janet and Mom and Dad today, and I know that 1999 will be an excellent year with its fair share of challenges. Thank you, dear Lord, for watching over my loved ones for yet another year. Please keep my powerful guardian angels looking out for them day and night. Amen!

---

2 January 1999

I slept in until 0800hrs this morning and as a result feel somewhat better than I did yesterday. My nose is still running, and I continue to have a hacking cough – just the kind of symptoms that patients want to see in their treating physician.

We had a very busy day clinically, and while very rewarding, it is also tiring when you never seem to get a break. This whining from the man who has just returned from four days of R&R is definitive proof that weakness has indeed taken root in my body. I spent half of my afternoon dealing with young men of around Nathan's age who are concerned that they may be going home with a "gift" from one of the girls whose acquaintance they made while on leave. The lads think the whole issue is very funny until I pull out the chlamydia swab and tell them, "I will have to insert this about two and a half inches up your penis." Believe me, they are in a very sober mood from that point on. These lads claim to have an awful lot of condom failures, and from my personal observation, it isn't because of their impressive physical endowment.

I found out today that the 3 RCR has a very large number of the Airborne soldiers who were with the 3 Commandos before that regiment was disbanded. These fellas are easy to spot because they usually have multiple tattoos, and at least one of the tattoos is of some paratrooping significance. The general public naively thinks the Canadian Airborne Regiment no longer exists. All that has happened is that the CAF has taken the regiment and spread it throughout all the other Army units.

We were informed today that if our fuel truck drivers had waited for two more seconds to jump from their vehicle they would have gone over the cliff, and we would likely have had to conduct two more funeral services.

Four of the ASC staff will be redeploying back to Canada tomorrow afternoon, and they aren't too hard to pick out of a crowd. They seem to exude a certain joie de vivre that those of us who are still a long way from going home are incapable of. This will be a difficult month, as I will be saying goodbye to so many people I have come to know and re-spect. On the other hand, it will be interesting to meet all the incoming rookies. The AOR remains generally quiet, and we all hope that it stays this way for at least another month.

---

3 January 1999

Only thirty days until I get to head home for good. I hope the time continues to fly by as fast as it did for the month of December. I managed to go to bed early last night and got about nine hours of good sleep. This was important because this morning six of us went off into the hills and did a one hour, thirty-five-minute run. Given my struggle with the flu-like weakness that has invaded my aging Air Force body, I am truly surprised how good I felt. This course has an eighteen-minute hill on it, and by the end of the ascent my legs felt like they weighed a ton. It is really nice to have some company for these sessions.

Yesterday the military police conducted their annual "Jail and Bail" campaign to raise money to pay for a stove for the school in Cazin. To send someone to jail, all you have to do is pay ten Deutsche Marks and fabricate various heinous crimes that they are alleged to have committed. The MPs then arrive on the doorstep of the person you fingered, read them their rights, arrest them and then drag them off to stand in front of a kangaroo court. As luck would have it, I was arrested late in the day and charged with shirking my duties, malingering, and failing to pay sufficient attention to the precious EpiNATO statistics (an annoying database that we have to maintain of all the injuries and illnesses that occur every week in our contingent). These were nothing but outrageous, malicious and unfounded lies, but despite all my pleading, they still hauled me off to the Crowbar Hotel.

It was obvious from the moment I entered the courtroom that the judge and his entire staff were incompetent, biased and totally corrupt – much like the actual Bosnian legal system. I was provided a defence counsel who was even dumber looking than the judge, and after he told the court that the accusations against me were entirely false, I decided to take matters into my own hands. I threw myself on the mercy of the court by shamelessly grovelling at the judge's feet and pleading for leniency. When I returned to my seat, the judge asked if I had anything further to say, so I requested my counsel to ask the judge if he had been working out lately because he sure was looking marvellous. It seems this was the straw that broke the camel's back; I was fined fifty Deutsche Marks or twenty minutes in jail. I selected incarceration and promptly phoned the medical staff to come and help bail me out. They ran over immediately, but rather than contributing a cent to my liberation, they elected to taunt me from afar. I was even denied my right to a conjugal visit. In the end, I managed to negotiate my freedom for twenty Deutsche Marks provided I gave the judge my camouflaged condom. It was all good fun, and the MPs ended up making enough money to buy the school a refrigerator and a stove. Hooah!

---

4 January 1999

The weather continues to be very mild here, and we are walking around in a sea of mud puddles. It's a good thing I have my platform combat boots.

I spent the morning in the Todorovo walk-in clinic, and it was a bit of a zoo. We had previously brought a bunch of clothing and shoeboxes to give to the kids, and I think that the locals have started to catch on. The clinic has virtually no heat, and we spent four hours seeing thirty-five patients with a wide assortment of odd maladies. Almost everyone comes expecting to receive a pill to cure their troubles, and some must be very disillusioned when the Western doctors don't have an all-powerful pharmaceutical to heal them. It seemed that every second person has had headaches for the last ten years or was suffering from stomach discomfort.

The population of this town is entirely Muslim, and they are currently in the middle of a holy period known as Ramadan, during which they must fast from dawn to dusk. I suspect that this is the cause of many of these people's headaches and abdominal discomforts. The Bosnian nurses were a little upset with me because I was taking too long to examine the patients, and they wanted to know why I wasn't as fast as the Canadian doctor from VK. I ignored them and carried on at my own pace. Working at Todorovo is a frustrating experience. They often do not have the exact medication I would like to use, and I doubt that the people I recommended be referred to see medical specialists will ever have this happen. The bottom line is that you do what you can and hope that it makes a difference in someone's life.

Upon returning to camp, I had two consults and a medical to do. By the time these were completed, the average soldier's working day was done, but I still had to do my medical advisor duties. I guess that is why it is 2230hrs, and I am still in my office working on this journal note.

As I predicted, despite the completion of Op Shoebox, Canadians have continued to send gifts, and we were just informed that another one thousand shoebox gifts have arrived in theatre. This is going to be interesting.

------

5 January 1999

If the weather is any indication, it is spring in the Box. It was sunny and very warm today – in fact so warm that people went running in T-shirts and shorts this afternoon. Our running group ran twice today. The fifty-minute morning run was very fast, and I must admit that the three days of diarrhea that I have been enjoying have left me feeling less than peppy. The afternoon run was a rare *célébration du soleil* and the best that I could do was drag my butt around the route without collapsing.

Apparently, someone decided to celebrate New Year's in a small town near Prijedor by detonating a bomb that destroyed the town's community complex. This is the second bombing that has occurred in this town, and it would appear that someone is trying to make a point – what exactly that point is, no one is sure.

The slagging continues – today the lads at the UMS decided to take my eating utensils and either wrap them up in sterile sheets or autoclave them and seal them in sterile packaging. I had no idea this had taken place until I went to lunch and pulled my eating equipment out of my utensils bag. Initially, I thought I had someone else's bag but quickly came to realize that I had been had. The lads seemed to love pulling one over on me, and I will now have to figure out how to slag them in retribution for their heinous crimes against my person.

Amazingly, we have managed to distribute the one thousand additional shoeboxes that we didn't know were coming. I am afraid that there may be more where those came from. Please Lord, could you turn the tap off on Op Shoebox.

I was just informed that all members of the ASC staff will have a two-day post-deployment retreat in Jasper in early April 1999. The spouses are funded to attend this event, which is aimed at allowing personnel an opportunity to work through any issues that may arise post-deployment. Given the close working relationship that I enjoy with this staff, the CO of the ASC had asked permission for me to attend this retreat, and it was approved. I hope that Janet will be allowed to go so we can spend a few days with our western relatives.

---

6 January 1999

The spring-like weather continues, and people here say that it is quite unusual for this area of the world and this time of the year.

Every day of this weather is one less day of winter that we have to endure. Life here is getting somewhat more comfortable for me but it does have its inconveniences, and when these occur, they remind you of the reality that you are not back in Canada. This week our e-mail server crashed several times. When this happens, I usually lose whatever document that I had been working on. The generator for the entire camp failed two nights ago, leaving us without power for nearly two hours. This occurred at 2300hrs and so only a few of us were aware it had even happened. If the power had been off longer and the weather had been much colder, it could have been very unpleasant.

Yesterday, I picked up my laundry, but it was still very damp. I guess all the melting snow created a leak somewhere, and my bag was the lucky recipient of a second cold-water rinse. I simply spread my damp clothing all over my humble sea container to air dry. If you expect five-star hotel treatment here, you are in for a major disappointment. With less than four weeks to go, it is amazing how many soldiers who ate well and didn't do much physical exercise throughout our deployment are now flooding into the gym to try and shed some deployment lard before they reunite with their spouse or partner. This sudden change in behaviour will likely result in many of them returning home with unwanted injuries.

Tomorrow morning, I will be flying to Banja Luka for a meeting of all the medical personnel in the Multinational Division Southwest. When we were originally informed that our flight request was approved, we were scheduled to be flying on "Mad Dog." This is the call sign for the only Czech helicopter that hasn't crashed and killed everyone in the last year. Considering the Czechs' dismal flight safety record, no one wants to fly in this bird, and that includes yours truly. I mentioned to the CO of the ASC my trepidation and that I would be asking my guardian angels to protect us on departure and return flights. Less than five minutes after I made this promise, the phone rang and we were informed that for some unknown reason, the flight schedules had been changed and we would now be travelling in a Canadian Griffon. Thank you for looking out for us, Lord.

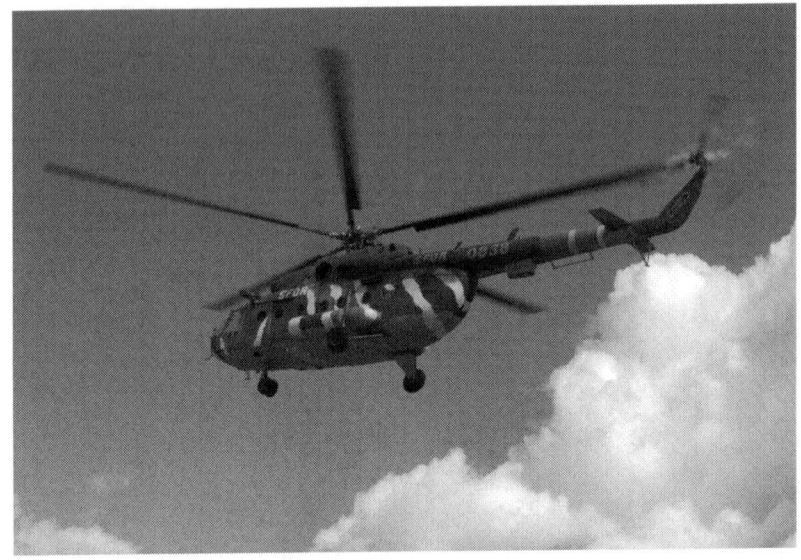

**A Czech Hip helicopter – given their extremely poor flight safety
record I was very grateful I never had to fly in one.**

---

7 January 1999

Today was yet another adventure here in Bosnia. We had a meeting
with the Division medical staff and were able to fly to and from Banja
Luka. We took off at 1000hrs and flew to Drvar to drop off the CO of
the Battle Group and several others for a pow wow of some sort. The
flight was forty minutes long and took us over mountains and along
narrow river canyons. The scenery was a mixture of absolute breathtaking beauty and shocking devastation. At one moment, we would
be flying over a turquoise-blue river, and on the other side of the next
hill we would fly over mile after mile of homes that were blown to
rubble. Somebody must have really wanted to blow up some of these

places because many of them were a long way off the beaten path. You sure get a unique perspective from the air. The area is littered with sinkholes, and nobody knows exactly what has caused them.

Our visit to Banja Luka was rather frustrating in that everyone there is relatively new, and so the CO of the ASC and I had to endure an afternoon of hearing things that we learned six months ago. We did get a tour of the Sea King helicopter that is used by the IRT (immediate response team). It is a pretty slick piece of equipment that has unfortunately been used far too often during this tour. The high point for me was skipping lunch and going to the regimental kit shop to buy a Norwegian fleece top and then spending half an hour buying black-market CDs. I was able to buy twenty-two great CDs, some of which were double albums, and they all cost the equivalent of five Canadian dollars. Now that's what I call a great deal.

We then spent ninety minutes waiting for our helicopter to return to take us home and were beginning to worry that we might be stranded there for the night. Our bird finally arrived at dusk, and by the time it was refueled it was nearly pitch-black, so the pilots had to fly using NVG (night vision goggles). These little babies amplify the minutest amount of light and allow the flight crew to see nearly as clearly as they can during the day. The first half of our flight was through the Republic of Srpska, and today is their Orthodox Christmas Day. For some perverse reason, these people celebrate any significant event – such as weddings, birthdays and Christmas – by firing their weapons into the air. Prior to take off, we were hearing gunshot reports from all around the airfield. When we were airborne, we could see streams of tracer rounds being fired on every side of our helicopter. It sure gives you a warm fuzzy feeling to know that if any one of these bullets happened to hit our helicopter in just the right place, we would fall out of the sky like a rock. We were hoping that the shooters weren't actually aiming for us.

At this evening's briefing, someone announced that their replacement would be arriving in one week, and his name was Capt Neil Armstrong. This raised a few eyebrows. When my turn came, I decided to continue my role as a mischief-maker and announced that my replacement, LCol John Glenn, would be here on the 29th. Once again, I was fortunate that everyone thought this was funny.

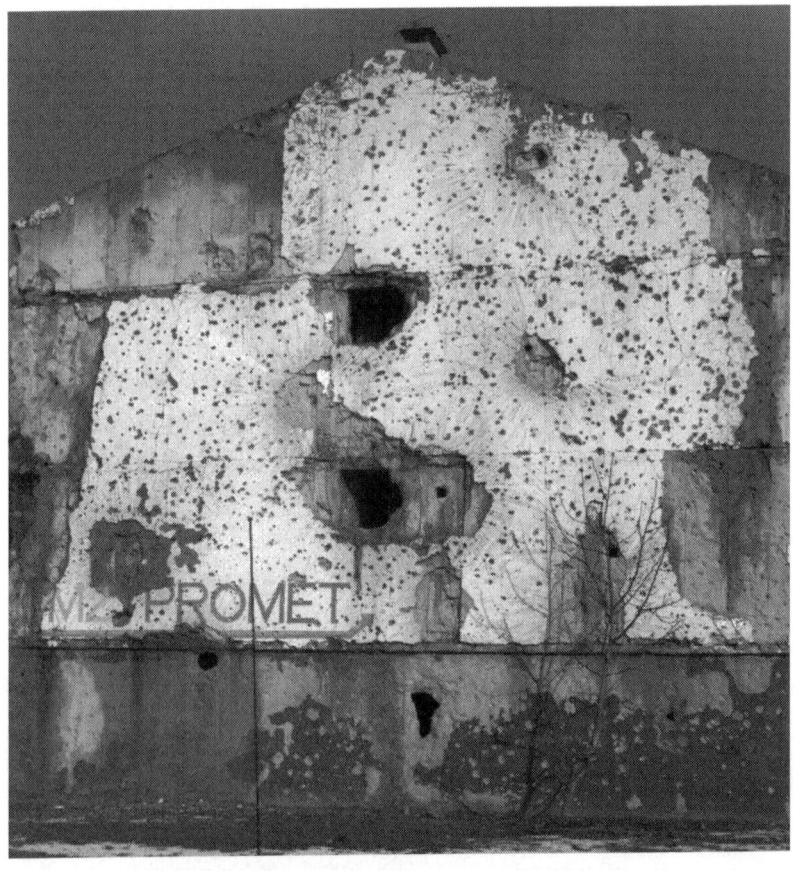

**A typical example of the destruction you would see travelling around
our area of responsibility in Bosnia.**

8 January 1999

This has been another extremely full day here in the fun capital of the world. It started off with a fast fifty-minute run with Captain Edora, and today it was me who was feeling peppy for a change. I then drove to VK for the Commander's weekly meeting. The atmosphere in the room these days is one of quiet confidence. That mood is soon likely to be shattered with the arrival of the rookies.

I met with Dr. Begovic and an American military physician and gave them a guided tour of both VK and Coralici. They were here for several reasons, not the least of which was the fact that the United States is substantially cutting back the size of their medical team at COM Z HQ in Zagreb, and as a result they will have nowhere to take their patients for dental care, x-rays, blood work or hospital admission. Without hesitation, we told the physician that we would be happy to see their personnel at no cost to them. Our American colleague found this hospitality difficult to comprehend until we explained that this is how we are currently operating with every other nation in theatre. This is not how the Americans normally function – they typically seem to want to remain self-sufficient. They departed at 1720hrs, and that left me with a whole twenty-five minutes to myself before having to board a bus that would take us to the Battle Group officers' goodbye dinner.

It turned out to be a very nice evening with a multi-course meal. The dinner was followed by a roasting of all the officers who were not part of the 3 RCR but supported them during this deployment. When it came to saying goodbye to the Three Amigos, they referred to us as "the Psycho, the Legal Beagle and the Quack." Guess which one I was. I must admit that the master of ceremonies was very kind to me – he took a couple of shots, but with the amount of ammunition I provided them during the tour, he could have spent the entire evening roasting me alone. As a token of their appreciation, they gave all three of us a commemorative print of the Battle Group's time here in Bosnia.

This will be a nice reminder of this time that I have been privileged to serve with them.

I do not know what is going on with the phones, but I have not been able to reach Janet for two days now. This is frustrating, as I would sure like to hear her voice.

---

9 January 1999

This morning as I was sauntering off to breakfast, I was informed that our alert status had changed, and so I had to go back and change into something less comfortable. Our status was listed as Black Alpha 2, which means that we must wear our helmets, flak vests and load-bearing vests, and carry our weapons in camp. It also means that we must travel in convoys of a minimum of two vehicles and have a long-barrelled weapon in every vehicle. This change has occurred for several reasons that I cannot disclose. It may also be related to the fact that French SFOR troops just killed a Serbian war criminal, and we are expecting reprisals. The entity armed forces in the Bosnian region are getting a little too cocky for their own good, and over the next while we will likely see SFOR put them firmly in their place. We cannot afford to let the entity armed forces do whatever they want, or we will surely see a return of full-blown ethnic violence. We are not even allowed to run inside our camp in this alert state.

The new ASC staff arrived in camp this evening, and the alert state had a few of them wide-eyed. I hope we didn't look as green as they look, when we first started working here. The new staff will have to learn fast, as the BG is entering what I am guessing will be a busy operational period, so they will have to be ready to function as well as the experienced ASC has.

I have spent the better part of the afternoon feeling somewhat frustrated at the way the BG continues to do business. The second half of this afternoon's operational briefing was highly secretive, and I was asked to leave while they had our junior BG medical officer remain. I don't think I am anyone special but the reason for my frustration is that, as the Commander's medical advisor, it is hard to give good advice when you don't know critical details about what is going on. I do not know why the BG can't seem to understand this, but you can bet they will come running for help when the brown stuff hits the fan.

I forgot to mention that at yesterday's dinner we were not allowed to drink any alcohol, and so all of the toasts were done with Kool-Aid served in wine glasses. I understand that there are policies to be followed, but you sure feel childish toasting the Queen with a cup of Freshie in your hand.

---

10 January 1999

With our increased security status, I was once again forbidden from running inside the camp today. I managed to run the fifty metres it takes to get to the gym and then spent seventy soul destroying minutes running on a treadmill. I absolutely hate running on a treadmill – I am pretty sure that I would give up running if this was the only way I was able to stay fit.

Our church service was another great experience for me, and I would think it was similarly great for everyone else in attendance. The celebrations are small and very personal, and we even had group discussions during the sermon. I will miss this aspect of being in theatre. Our little makeshift chapel is a mosaic of religious materials from all over Canada, and this serves to make it a very special place.

This afternoon, we had our long-anticipated medal parade at the castle in VK. It was a small ceremony, with twenty-three of us receiving our NATO decorations from Col Natynczyk. The colonel also handed out his commendations to the soldiers whose performance was exceptional in some way. Our two administrative clerks and our public affairs officer were each presented with a Commander CCSFOR Commendation. The G4, Capt Horlock, was awarded a DCDS Commendation that comes with both a plaque and a decoration that worn as part of the dress uniform. All four were deserving of recognition, and it was nice to see them acknowledged in front of their peers.

Following the parade, we were treated to what can only be described as the most elaborate and hands-down best feast I have ever attended. Each table setting had twenty-one utensils, and there were seven servings before we got to the main course. The entrees included escargot, lobster Newberg and quiche lorraine. The main course

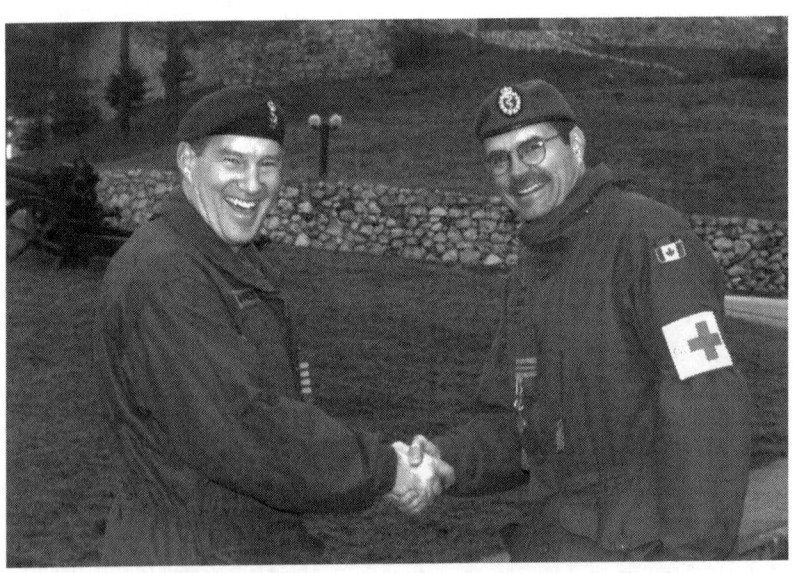

Receiving my NATO Service Medal for the Former Yugoslavia from Col. Natynczyk who would later go on to be the Chief of Defence Staff. I could not have asked for a better boss.

had five different filet mignons and was followed by three additional courses. In total the meal lasted four hours, and I was gastronomically quite uncomfortable due to the volume and variety of the food that was served. It was nice to share a special meal with people you have worked so hard with for so long. You can feel the excitement building for our impending return home.

---

11 January 1999

Despite yesterday's gluttony, I was able to struggle through my typical morning run without throwing up on myself or any of my running buds.

I spent the morning in the UMS because Captain Edora was covering the Todorova clinic. It was nice to be working with the medical staff again, and we even performed some minor surgery on a soldier's face. I do like cutting out lumps and bumps and would love to work in a clinic that specialized in this type of work.

This afternoon, I loaded my unaccompanied baggage onto a Medium Logistic Vehicle Wheeled (MLVW) and drove it up to VK for the big check-in that was supposed to take only six minutes. I must admit, I was somewhat skeptical that the Army was capable of such efficiency, and as it turns out, my doubting Thomas attitude was not ill-founded. The whole process ended up requiring seventy-five minutes and involved the usual production of forms in quadruplicate. For some unknown reason, I seem to be a living nightmare for the administrative folks handling these assembly lines. Not only was I bringing all of my kit at one time, but I was also bringing three boxes when everyone else was entitled to only two. My kit ended up weighing fifty pounds more than we are each entitled to, and I was the only person in the contingent with an Australian military-issue battle box that is twice the size of the standard CAF issue. Despite having warned them that this is what I would be arriving with, the first question they asked me was if I was aware that I was checking in baggage in excess of my entitlement. This response is so consistent it is almost comical, and I have learned to just roll with the punches. It didn't take long for everything to finally get straightened out, and I was eventually on my way.

Saying goodbye to most of my worldly possessions is just another reminder that I will soon be heading home to my family. I am struggling not to get overly excited yet because I still have a whole lot of last-minute things to do around here.

The old ASC staff are busy bringing the new ASC staff up to speed, and while the former are definitely happy people, the new ASC personnel look a little overwhelmed. It won't be long before they are in charge, and their learning curve will be very steep.

Only twenty-two more days till I get to hold my wife and kids in my arms again. Please keep them safe, dear Lord.

---

12 January 1999

It has once again been a very full day, but I find that the closer I get to D-Day (departure day), the more mellow I am becoming. The weather here continues to be spring-like, and our running team swelled to eight nutcases this morning.

Captain Edora spent the entire day giving redeployment stress debriefings that every soldier in theatre is required to receive. These debriefings are aimed at getting soldiers to mentally prepare for reintegrating back into their families and their old jobs. The emphasis of these sessions is on basic issues such as discussing your feelings with your spouse not automatically criticizing any changes they may have made while you were away and telling your family that you love and missed them. While the messages were very simple, they are extremely important because many soldiers experience problems reintroducing themselves back into their families after having been gone for nearly a year. I think my family and my fellow headquarters co-workers should get this debriefing as they may have trouble adjusting to the return of the battle-hardened, combat-ready, weakness-rejecting, fighting machine that I have become.

While Captain Edora was doing the debriefings, I spent my day seeing patients again, and that was fine by me. I got to supervise one of our medical assistants while he removed a dermatofibroma (a skin lesion) from a patient today, and he did a superb job. He seemed to enjoy the responsibility and was very happy when I assured him that I could not have done any better.

The new ASC staff will start working the wards tomorrow, and this is when the real learning will begin. Apparently, we are sending a second ASC to the Congo sometime soon, and both our surgeon and our Sleepy Doc are very disappointed that they are serving in Bosnia, while their colleagues will be going somewhere new and exciting. Given the shortage of specialist medical officers we have in the CAF and the number of taskings going on throughout the world, our surgeon and anaesthetist may find themselves replacing themselves on the next rotation – wouldn't that be a morale booster.

Speaking of morale boosters, our lawyer managed to arrange to head home five days early, and NDHQ reached him today to tell him that he will be required to attend a conference in Ottawa the day after he returns to Canada. Can you imagine spending seven months away from your family only to be told you won't have any downtime when you return to Canada. It is little wonder that soldiers get disgruntled when they are shown so little respect.

13 January 1999

A gigantic blob of weakness must have landed on the camp last night because when I went to the front gate to run this morning, I was all by myself. This was quite a contrast from the day before and quite a disappointment because it meant that I once again had the privilege of running around in small circles behind a barbed wire fence. I made a point of questioning the courage of all my running companions I happened to meet as I went about my daily business. I did this to ensure they understood how much I didn't appreciate being totally abandoned this morning.

Once again, I had a clinically busy morning, which is wonderful. The new ASC staff are starting to get settled in their new jobs, and this means that things sure get crowded. At times, the staff are almost tripping over each other. I briefed the incoming CO of the ASC on issues that I feel she needs to be concerned about, and it is obvious she is experiencing the same information overload that swamped us all in the very beginning. I only hope that before I leave, she and her staff will feel a great deal more comfortable with their important role in theatre.

Major Livingstone has never been a commanding officer before, and I am sure the Army will be testing her out very early on. I have warned her about this and encouraged her to stand her ground, or she will have nothing but headaches.

The surgeon has indicated that he does not want to do any surgery at the Bihac hospital, which in my opinion is not a good decision. If things are going well, our surgical team does not have the opportunity to do much surgery in our ASC, and so the only way to stay sharp is to do surgical procedures at the local hospitals. This seems to have been a big morale booster for the previous Canadian surgical teams, and if the surgeon takes this away, ASC personnel are likely to experience a very long, boring tour. I hope that he changes his mind.

I have been listening to my new CDs while I work in the office, and I must say they are great. I enjoy this so much that I am thinking of bringing my ghetto blaster and CDs with me when I return to work at NDMC.

It is time to call it a night, as I need to rest up to kick the butts of my running buds tomorrow morning.

14 January 1999

Our entire contingent seems to have come down with a viral illness that causes robust coughing, a sore throat, congestion and a runny nose. Now that I have finally begun recovering from this illness, I have decided to attribute this outbreak to the "Weakness Plague." It really has affected a great number of our soldiers, and it shows no signs of slowing down. It is also hard to prevent these types of infections when we are all living and working in such close quarters.

Today, I had the true privilege of going to the ranges with "Those of Whom We Dare Not Speak" to fire weapons that no one else is allowed to use. They will neither confirm nor deny that I was ever there, so you will just have to take my word for it. This opportunity transpired after I asked their sergeant major when the Secret Squirrels would be shooting next. I told him that Captain Clifford is a gun nut, and an opportunity to shoot with the Grey Men would likely be the highlight of his life. When the sergeant major confirmed that Captain Clifford could come out with them, he also invited me to come along. Woo-hoo! So off we went to the range: a pair of docs, the two Grey Men, the "go bang toys" and several thousand rounds of ammunition. I must admit that it was a real hoot to fire all these weapons. We both had the opportunity to use the MP5 assault machine gun, the modified C8 fully automatic rifle, the modified C9 and a special handgun. They were all great to use, but hands down the weapon I enjoyed firing the most was the MP5. At ten metres, I could hit a Styrofoam cup over and over again. In fact, I don't think I missed on a single shot, and I actually started trying to hit the piece of string that the cups were suspended from. The MP5 is lightweight, easy to handle, very small and deadly accurate. These are the reasons virtually all the special forces in the world use it as their close-quarters weapon of choice. All told, I got to fire off about 350 rounds, and that is likely more rounds than I have had a chance to fire throughout my entire military career. I was quite excited about this experience, and I think the operators are beginning to worry that I might be a commando wannabe. Hooah! Hooah!

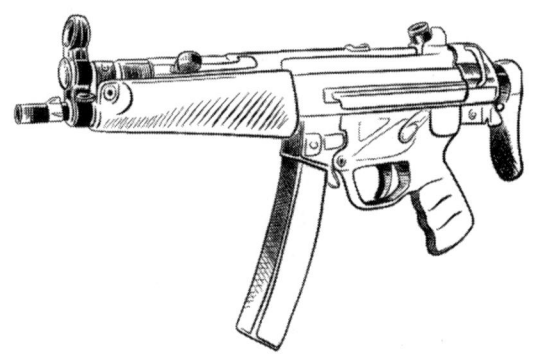

The MP5 Submachine Gun

15 January 1999

I will remember today for a very long time, as it is the first time in my life that I was able to crack off a one-arm push-up. While we were waiting for a meeting, someone asked me to perform a push-up. I asked what type they wanted, and of course they asked for the one-arm version. I warned the group that despite months of working on this skill, I have only been able to go down without smashing my face into the ground, but once safely on the ground I have not been able to push myself back up no matter how hard I try. Today when I went down and tried to push back up, to my complete amazement my body began to rise off the ground, and before I knew it my right arm was fully extended. I realize that in the annals of human achievement this insignificant moment is the equivalent of a mouse farting in Saskatchewan. However, it was something I had dedicated a lot of effort to, and I think working on some kind of non-military goal during a deployment is a valuable distraction from the abnormal world we are living in.

The new ASC staff ran the show independently for the first time today, and what they lack in experience they are making up for in enthusiasm. On their first day, they were blessed with a visit from Brigadier-General Menzies who will soon be the Surgeon General for the British Armed Forces. The staff ran around the entire morning preparing for his arrival, working on the misguided premise that he would arrive precisely as scheduled at 1300hrs. I did warn them that this was highly unlikely to occur, and sure enough, he arrived an hour earlier than planned, and everyone was in a complete panic. I chose to spend my waiting time knotting a paracord tail for someone's Gerber tool.

As part of his tour, General Menzies was shown the inside of a Bison ambulance. While he was sitting in the ambulance, one of the medical assistants opened the roof hatch to show him how it worked. When the hatch was lifted, the good general was showered by a deluge of water. It was embarrassing for the medical assistant, but to his credit the general took this unscheduled shower in stride. While he and his staff were visiting the UMS, one of his nursing officers asked our driver, who happens to be an infantry soldier, what kind of training he gets. This fellow has a great sense of humour and responded that he first learned how to start IVs and suture people up. Once he mastered these basic skills, he progressed to doing neurosurgery and then was posted to Bosnia. She bought everything he told her hook, line and sinker. I am sure our British colleagues now believe we have a neurosurgeon in theatre that we have been hiding from them.

It has come to my attention that the new ASC team has a collection of very young and good-looking women. It is very funny to watch the infantry sharks circling the ASC in the hopes of some end-of-tour romance. Good luck lads!

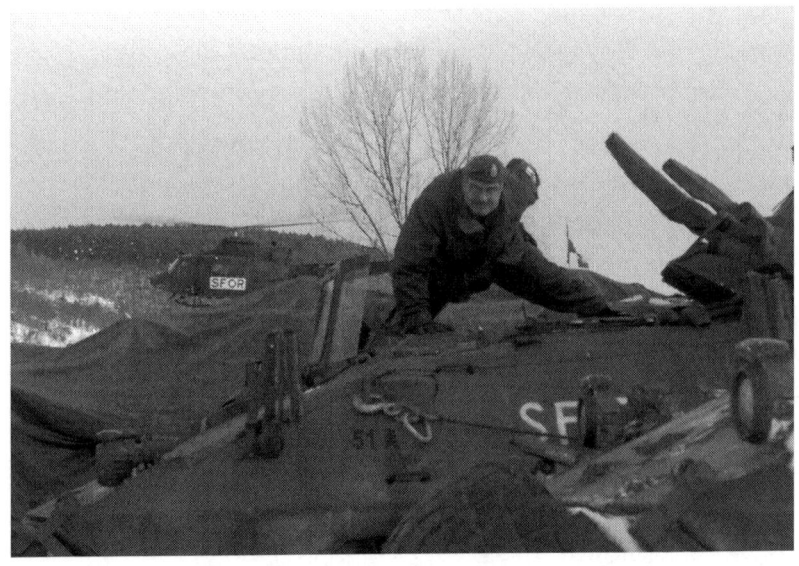

Me showing off after I was finally able to do the elusive one-armed push up – what a goof!

---

16 January 1999

The transfer of authority between the ASC for Roto 3 and Roto 4 officially occurred this morning. This involved a small ceremony where the Commander of CCSFOR witnessed the outgoing and incoming commanding officers sign over power. This ceremony was somewhat sad to watch as it meant that in four short hours I would be saying farewell to eighteen people that I have enjoyed working and playing with for the last six months. At the same time, it was very exciting for the new ASC staff because they are now officially on their own and calling all the shots. I am certain there will be many changes, and I will need to sit back and help out only when appropriate. This could be a challenge as I'm sure I will instinctively want to rush in and rescue them. For their sakes, I hope that this ASC team gets a slower introduction to major medical challenges than the crew of Roto 3 did.

The combination of great weather and the fact that we will all soon be heading home has left Stalag Coralici in a relatively mellow mood. This is probably a good thing because everyone is tired of working day and night trying to stay focused on our mission.

It appears that tales of my legendary skills weaving parachute cord have begun to spread far and wide. This afternoon as I was walking around the camp, an older soldier stopped me and asked if I would teach him how to weave a Gerber tail. I tried not to show my surprise and agreed to begin lessons the next time we ran into each other. With any luck, this could turn out to be that second career I've been looking for.

The two new specialists are extremely unhappy at having to come here again, and unfortunately, they are taking every opportunity to tell this to anyone who will listen. I fear that the new CO of the ASC is going to have her hands full dealing with this issue, and it could make her tour much more difficult than it needs to be.

The old ASC staff drove off in a bus at 1300hrs, and they sure looked happy to be heading home to their friends and loved ones. I am getting excited too but will try and control myself until my replacement arrives in camp. It sure will be nice to hug my family once again. Lord, please continue to look after them for me.

17 January 1999

Today was an absolutely gorgeous spring-like day. The sun was shining, it was warm, and virtually all the snow has melted. Today's workout had us running the mountainous club route, and both the footing and scenery were outstanding.

We had the last of the Commander's monthly conferences today, and it ran quite long. Everyone seemed quite impressed that I somehow managed to remain awake for the whole thing – a bit of a miracle I must admit. The meeting was informative in the sense that it outlined a number of very interesting issues. Since Roto 3 has been in theatre, we have put forward for and acquired foreign funding for forty-three community reconstruction projects worth DM1.8 million. This is a huge contribution. Our drivers will have covered nearly four million kilometres and experienced only fifty-eight motor vehicle accidents, the vast majority of which were not our fault. This operation has cost the Canadian people $15.6 million over and above all our salaries and benefits. We have sent a total of sixty-one personnel home earlier than expected – twenty of them were medical repatriations, and three were in coffins. Sadly!

According to information relayed during the conference, things in Bosnia and Kosovo are once again beginning to heat up. This week, authorities discovered an open grave with the bodies of fifty recently slaughtered Kosovars. With the snow rapidly melting away, it won't be long before full-blown war breaks out. In Bosnia, SFOR continues to apprehend war criminals, and there are still plenty of these sons of bitches out there. Every time we capture one, it triggers a flurry of threats against SFOR and the United Nations International Police Task Force. Since the New Year, SFOR soldiers have been physically accosted, and in one incident they were told face to face that if they captured any more war criminals, they would all be shot, and their interpreter hanged. The sad thing is that given the atrocities these people committed on their neighbours, we know they wouldn't think twice about killing some SFOR soldiers.

Today I heard a new military acronym being used. Someone asked what we were going to do about a certain problem, and the response they received was "RFP." We all looked around with question marks on our faces and someone finally explained that it stands for "Roto Four problem"! As we get closer and closer to heading home, I think this mentality will become more and more prevalent.

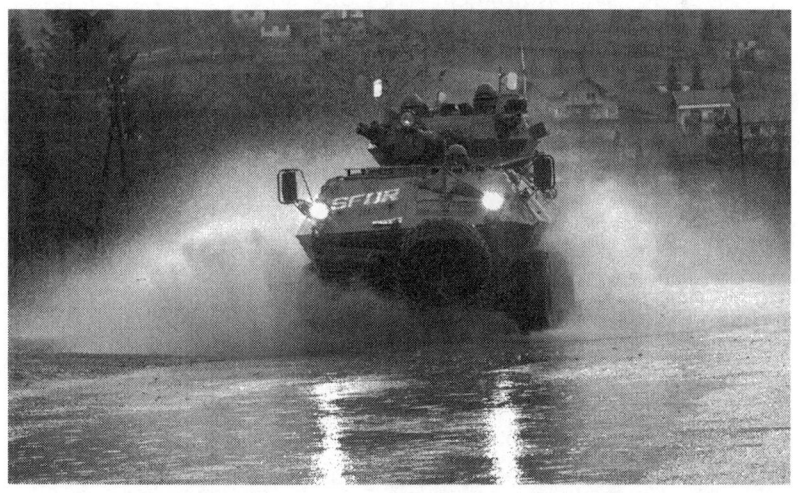

A Cougar vehicle covering some of those four million kilometers that of our soldiers travelled during our deployment to keep the peace in Bosnia.

---

18 January 1999

The amazing weather here continues to hold – it will be a major letdown when the temperatures finally return to their seasonal norm.

I think the folks of Roto 3 are in for a real shock when we finally land back in Canada because it is still very much winter in that part of the world.

I had the scare of my life last night when I finally took off my uniform. Earlier in the day we left the camp for the Commander's conference, and therefore had to have our weapons with us. I remember clearing my weapon when we returned to camp. However, this evening when I removed my holster, I noticed that it was extremely light, and to my complete horror, my 9mm pistol wasn't in it. This is a very, very, very serious problem. I cannot overstate how grave a sin it is in the military to lose your weapon in a theatre of war, especially if you happen to be a senior officer. After we returned to camp, I recalled escorting our vehicle to its parking spot, and the route I walked took us right past the military police building. I could not shake the sickening feeling that one of our police officers found my pistol laying in the snow when he was heading to the Mess for a doughnut. I quickly retraced my steps, and I could feel a sense of panic building as I failed to find any evidence of my pistol. The only other possibility was that it fell out of my holster when I was sitting in the ASC's Iltis vehicle. When I opened the door to the passenger's side there was still no evidence of my missing pistol, so I slid my hand between the seat and the door panel. Words cannot express the relief I felt when my

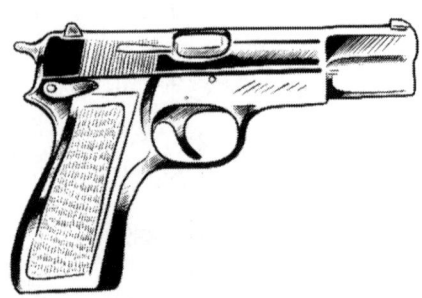

My long lost 9mm pistol

fingers touched the cold butt of my missing weapon. I have no idea how I did not hear something that heavy striking the vehicle's metal floor when it fell out of my holster. Thank God it was there and that I didn't have to alert the military police. If this had been necessary, all hell would have broken loose, and while I don't know what would have happened to me, I guarantee it would not have been pretty. I think I will tie a lanyard to my weapon so that a little disaster like this can never happen again.

I somehow injured my left hip and was forced to walk this morning's workout. While I did enjoy getting off the camp for some exercise, walking just doesn't feel as nice as running. I hope this discomfort doesn't last for too long.

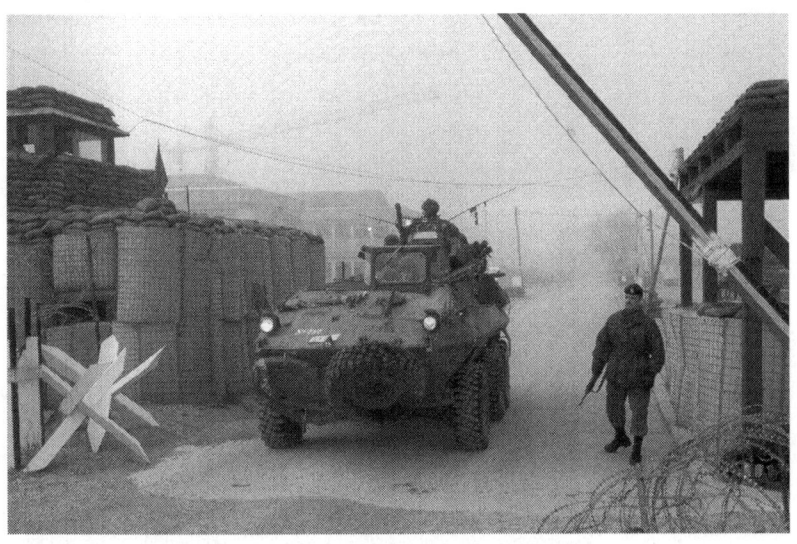

The front gate to all our camps were heavily guarded and every soldier was required to demonstrate they had no bullets in the firing chambers of their weapons. The army refer to this safety measure as proving your weapon.

The general mood in the camp is one of expectancy as everyone you meet these days is heading home really soon. The first crowd of Roto 3 personnel will be departing in four days' time, and it's only fifteen days for me. One of Nathan's friends, Wayne Richardson, will soon be arriving in theatre for his seven-month rotation. I do not envy his parents – I would not want any of my children working here. Watch over him, Lord, while he is deployed here. Amen!

---

19 January 1999

While the great weather here is cause for some of us to celebrate, it is the worst thing that could be happening for Kosovo. Our intelligence personnel indicate that the situation in Kosovo is rapidly worsening, and I am certain that all-out war will break out in the near future. If this happens, there will be thousands more dead before next winter, and many more will flee their country in the hopes of remaining alive. One of our nurses, a Med A (medical assistant) and I went out with one of Oscar Company's patrols this afternoon to meet a family of Kosovar refugees in this exact situation. This family of five – including three children four years old and younger – fled Kosovo with only two bags of personal belongings and the clothes on their backs. They are currently living in a home about forty-five minutes southwest of Coralici and have very little available to help them survive.

Similar to the previous Kosovar families we have helped, we found this family living in the only heated room in the house, which could not have been more than ten feet by ten feet. The soldiers brought them food, clothing, vitamins, bandages, cooking oil and friendship. I wish the anti-military press in our country could see the nobility of our soldiers doing this kind of work on their own initiative. They brought the medical team along because they were concerned that one of the children was ill. Apparently, the two-year-old child complains of joint and bone pains at night and has trouble sleeping. I examined the child thoroughly and the only thing I can conclude is that his discomforts may be caused by malnutrition. His mother did not breastfeed him, and they do not have access to milk or fresh fruits and vegetables. How can an infant build a healthy body without these essential building blocks? Luckily, we had some fresh fruit for them and a three-and-a-half-month supply of Flintstones Chewable Vitamins. The soldiers will look into bringing milk with them on their next visit. I also used this opportunity to present the family with homemade quilts made by the good folks of Russell, Ontario. I couldn't think of a better use for these gifts made by the loving hands of the women in my community.

I have been greatly moved by a number of soldiers who have been kind enough to tell me they will miss me because I seem to really care and take my time to treat them like real people. This was unexpected and makes me feel wonderful because this is how I think our military personnel should always be treated regardless of their rank.

I have been unable to get through on the phone to talk to Janet for several days now, and I really miss hearing her voice. Guardian angels of mine, please keep a very close watch over my loved ones. Amen.

---

20 January 1999

Only thirteen days until I get to go home to my family and friends. It seems so close, but there is a part of me that keeps saying, "Stay calm, big fella, you still have a ways to go yet." Two of the corporals from the UMS staff are leaving in two days, and they were almost drunk with joy for the entire day. Currently, the most-asked question in our camp is "So how many days do you have left?" The really cruel people knowingly ask this question of the recently arrived ASC staff, and then give a little laugh and walk away.

I finally managed to get to talk to Janet today, and she sounded fine until it was time for me to say goodbye because I was running out of my allotted phone time. Towards the end, I could hear her voice cracking, and I could tell she needed some hugs and kisses. It sure leaves you feeling helpless when you know your lover needs to be with you, and there is absolutely nothing you can do to be there for her. I only hope Janet knows that she and the children are the most important treasures in my life. This tour has been challenging for me, but I believe it was probably as much or more of a challenge for Janet. Hang in there my love, I will soon be home and messing everything up again.

It appears that the two ASC members who came on patrol with me yesterday enjoyed themselves so much, they have recommended these types of visits to all their colleagues. When I walked into the ASC this evening, I was immediately pounced on by a bunch of people who want to go on the next adventure with Dr. Darrell into the wilds of Bosnia. At least this time, our vehicle didn't break down, slide off the road, get into an accident or get lost in a minefield. It will be interesting to see just how keen this group remains when they have been here for six months.

The tempo of life in our camp has slowed to a near standstill, and this sure makes it easy to complete all those last-minute tasks one has to do before heading back home. This lull is only going to last a couple more days because the Roto 4 Battle Group advance party arrives on Friday. Watch out world, the rookies are coming.

---

21 January 1999

It is almost miraculous the way the good weather is holding in here. I still have been unable to run because my left hip continues to be sore, but today it was much less sore than it has been for the last five days. With any luck, this annoying injury will heal in the next few days.

Tomorrow morning, the first group of personnel from the Battle Group will be heading up to Zagreb to fly home. These folks sure seem happy to be leaving, and the good mood that they generate is quite infectious. I have been getting all my last-minute jobs taken care of and hopefully will be able to relax when my replacement finally arrives.

The 1 RCR Battle Group advance party will arrive in Coralici at 1600hrs tomorrow, and from then on I think we will watch the entire camp wind up once again. Happy, happy, joy, joy!

Two weeks ago, when I went to work at the clinic at Todorovo, I was accompanied by one of our medical assistants, Leading Seaman (LS) Tofts. We saw children with all kinds of diseases, including a case of chicken pox. Yesterday, he began to feel unwell in the morning, and by the evening he had broken out with a clear case of chicken pox. He sure looks miserable. We have confined him to his sea container so that he doesn't spread disease and pestilence throughout the camp. I made a house call this morning – technically it was a sea container call – and LS Tofts seems to be taking his ailment in stride. I have started referring to his sea container as "the leper colony," and his colleagues have nicknamed him "Fester." Unfortunately, we had to delay his flight back home until he is no longer contagious. I imagine this must be extremely disappointing for him.

This evening there was a group of four soldiers being given remedial drill on the parade square in front of the headquarters building. This type of punishment achieves several things for the Army. First, it embarrasses the soldiers who are forced to do the drill. Second, it tells everyone that these fellows did something wrong. Third, it serves as a deterrent for others who might be tempted to follow in their footsteps. I am told that these lads smuggled some beer into their platoon house, and they are going to get some heavy-duty fines to go along with their mandatory drill sessions.

We currently have a soldier in the ward who is suffering from a flare-up of ulcerative colitis. He is supposed to be heading home tomorrow, but I doubt that he will be well enough to safely travel. Not only is he likely to be delayed in arriving home to his wife and kids, but he is losing all the weight he worked so hard to put on in the camp's weight room. Lord, help him to feel well enough to fly home tomorrow.

---

22 January 1999

Our ill young man did not make it onto the plane this morning because he simply isn't well enough to travel. When I talked to him today, he was understandably frustrated but realizes that he isn't ready for the physical demands of the thirteen-hour flight back home. I have recommended to the surgeon that we have a medical team from Canada come over on the next flight and escort him home. The surgeon doesn't feel this is required, and it will be interesting to see who ends up having made the correct call.

I have noted that many soldiers have a distinct walk whereby they hold their arms away from their sides as though their latissimus dorsi muscles are so large that they simply cannot get their arms any closer to their bodies. This helps to create the illusion of hugeness. For the occasional soldier, this is the only way they can walk, while many others only fake it. In the wonderful world of military medicine, the fakers are said to suffer from "imaginary lat syndrome" (ILS). This comical condition isn't an exclusively military problem, and in fact can be found wherever there are insecure men who want to look bigger than they really are.

One of the soldiers who were charged last night received a $1,200 fine and seven days in jail. The ridiculous part about the jail sentence is that he will be going to jail in Petawawa, and by the time he finishes serving his seven days in prison, he will be home sooner than he would have been had he not been charged. Given the fabulous ambience at Stalag Coralici, I can't help wondering if he is being punished or rewarded.

When you are finished shooting at a military shooting range, everyone who participated must make a declaration to the range officer which goes like this: "I have no live rounds or empty cartridges in my possession, sir!" I learned another version of this declaration today, and it goes like this: "I have no live rounds or empty cartridges in my possession. I also have no mortars in my quarters, no bombs in my palms, no rockets in my pockets and no brass up my ass, sir!" I personally prefer the second version.

The advance party of 1 RCR arrived this afternoon – this camp is going to be a very crowded place for the next ten days. As odd as it may seem, I cannot help feeling somewhat resentful watching all these strange faces taking our camp from us.

---

23 January 1999

I had a great workout this morning, and my left hip hardly bothered me at all. I am enjoying doing more upper body work. Who knows, if I keep this up, I may even be able to do more than a single one-armed push-up at a time.

With everyone in the "I'm heading home" frame of mind, the demand for my medical services has really dropped off. I am very grateful that this was not the case for the majority of the tour, or I would have been a very unhappy camper. Instead of worrying about this steep decline in business, I have decided to relax a little and enjoy my last few weeks in theatre. The last thing I want to do is return home a burnt-out mess.

The soldiers here use a unique time-accounting system that seems to be aimed at creating the illusion that they have less time left to serve in theatre. For example, a soldier who has four days left to serve will often refer to this period as "three days and a wakie." The "wakie" refers to the day they will be travelling home. Somehow, three days and a wakie seems to sound so much better than four days. According to the Army time system, I currently have ten days and a wakie.

We have been told that the day we arrive in Petawawa, it may be too late at night for us to be processed by the Arrival Assistance Group (AAG). This means we will have the opportunity to spend a glorious night in quarters – wouldn't that just be the icing on the cake.

This afternoon I went for a fitness walk with three ladies from the ASC. When we were returning to the camp, we came upon a pair of dogs that were mating on the trail. As we came closer, the dogs became frightened and decided to move. I don't know how they did it, but the two dogs ended up pointed in opposite directions with their butts stuck together. The female dog was the larger of the two animals, and when she started to head away from us, she ended up dragging the poor male who was stuck inside her. The funniest part was when the pair hit a set of stairs, and she had to lift him off the ground to go up. This had to be painful, but after being dragged for about two minutes, the young male finally fell to his freedom. I doubt that many people ever get the opportunity to witness this comedy of nature.

I am not the most popular man with the ASC staff tonight because I insisted that we have a medical team from Canada sent over to assist our sick soldier during his strategic evacuation (STRATEVAC) back to Canada. Hopefully, when all the smoke settles this will turn out to be the right decision. Lord, watch over this young man so that we can return him safely to his young family. Amen.

24 January 1999

This morning I was able to run the majority of my workout, and I experienced no pain in my hip. This was very nice given that I was training on a very hilly course. In fact, the course was so hilly that when I reached the top there was dense fog and half a centimetre of frost coating absolutely everything. It truly was a beautiful sight.

With the influx of Roto 4 personnel, the new personnel are now using our beautiful chapel as transient quarters. Being flexible Christians, we held our Mass in the call sign eight office and it really was enjoyable. This experience demonstrates for me that the great cathedrals of the world that cost zillions of dollars to build are not required for a meaningful celebration of the Word of God. I have often thought that Jesus would have preferred the temple builders to invest their money into caring for the less fortunate.

This afternoon, two of the nursing officers and I went out on patrol with the boys of Oscar Company. They went all over the place, and while they had four families to visit, they repeatedly stopped along the roadside to give gift bags to the children who ran out when they saw us coming down the road. Two of the families we visited now have roofs on their homes because of the soldiers we were travelling with. For the other two families, it appears that our soldiers are their major source of food supplies. These soldiers are making a real difference here, and this was summed up so very eloquently by an old man who commented as he walked past our vehicle, "Canada goot!" Canada truly is a great country, and the vast majority of its soldiers are great ambassadors.

I sent an e-mail to the Chief of Medical Operations and the Surgeon General this evening. I expressed my concern that the Canadian Forces medical system has been diminished to the point that the medical team in theatre is having trouble ensuring that the patients we repatriate to Canada are well cared for. I told them exactly what I am witnessing here, but I have no idea how they will react. I guess if I am told that

I get to stay in Bosnia for another seven months, it will be a pretty good indication that they found my comments offensive. It wouldn't be the first time in my career that speaking truth to power didn't help me climb the food chain.

25 January 1999

Despite the fact that I ran a full workout for the first time in a week, today has undoubtedly been the most exasperating that I have spent in theatre to date. We appear to have cut back our CAF medical services to the point where patient care is going to be seriously compromised. Sending our patient back to Canada is proving to be more than our medical system can handle. As unbelievable as it may seem, we have spent nearly two full days trying to get an ambulance to meet our patient at the Ottawa airport and transport him to the Ottawa Civic Hospital.

At 2200hrs this evening, the CO of the ASC still did not have anyone who would provide a medical team to take our patient in the ambulance. The aeromedical evacuation team would not do it because they would be exceeding their maximum allowable work time. This was enough to make me spit fire. What the hell is this crap about a maximum work time? Are we not in the military where we get on with it until the job is done? NDMC has no beds, no ambulances and no medical crews to provide for the ambulances. It has become, for all intents and purposes, a completely useless administrative building that houses a whole bunch of medical people, many of which haven't seen a patient in so very long, they have forgotten what it's like for those of us who still do. The civilian medical authorities have no responsibility for the care of our soldier, and they won't even guarantee that our patient will have a bed in the Ottawa Civic Hospital. It appears that the medical staff from CFB Petawawa will have to come all the way to Ottawa to pick him up at the airport, and if there is no room available at the Civic Hospital, they will have to take him back to Petawawa where they also have no hospital bed for him.

We are trying to make these arrangements for one of the soldiers we sent into harm's way on Christmas Day when the Battle Group retook the Martin Brod region that Croatia had been illegally occupying. I have so many emotions churning inside me that it is distressing: I am frustrated, embarrassed, disappointed and angry all at the same time. I finally phoned NDMC at 2210hrs and told them that we were tired of dealing with this problem, and that not only was this unacceptable care for our soldiers, but it was total bullshit. This seemed to get the Lieutenant-Colonel's attention, and ten minutes later everything was miraculously worked out. It is very sad when this is what it takes to ensure that we are taking proper care of our ill and injured personnel. This disgraceful incident has demonstrated for me that the health care system in the CAF is in major trouble.

---

26 January 1999

The sun is beginning to come up earlier and earlier, which sure makes training in the morning a great deal more pleasant. There are more and more people running in the morning, and this is almost entirely the result of the new crew coming on board. I give them a month before their good fitness intentions will die just like they did for the majority of the soldiers that went before them. Weakness is everywhere!

Our sick soldier was not feeling well this morning, but we still managed to transport him by ambulance to Zagreb where he was loaded onto the airbus and taken back to Canada. A medical team from Canada was on the plane to care for him, and he will have a litter on which he can lay down and, hopefully, get some sleep. There is supposed to be an ambulance meeting him on the runway in Ottawa, and from there he will enter the world of civilian medicine where I no longer have any influence over what quality of care he is provided. I will just have to trust that all will go well. Please Lord, help our soldier not to suffer too much during his flight back home to his wife and children.

Captain Edora's replacement arrived today, and Fil is definitely a happy boy because he will soon head home to the loving arms of his new wife. I will miss him as a colleague, a friend, and a running and basketball bud. The ASC staff continue to settle in, and Stalag Coralici is rapidly becoming a place full of strangers. The one new person I did recognize was MCpl (Master Corporal) Jerry Conners who worked with Janet and me at the base hospital in Chatham, New Brunswick. He married one of the ladies who also worked in the base hospital, and they now have two little girls to call their own. He hasn't changed much – just a little less hair and a little larger pant size.

The Three Amigos will become the two amigos as of tomorrow when our lawyer leaves for Canada. I have enjoyed working with Sylvain and will always consider him my friend. I hope he feels the same way.

Time for bed, as I must be up early to travel to Zagreb. I am grateful that, this time, I will not be coordinating the return of the remains of a deceased soldier. Instead, I will be going to Zagreb to take part in the CAF site visit for this year's Conseil international du sport militaire (CISM) Military World Games which will be held in this beautiful city.

---

27 January 1999

It is now midnight, and I have just wrapped up shooting another episode of Nightmare Trip with Dr. Darrell. The weather here has been exceptional for over a month, and the one day I had to travel a long way by road, I awoke to rain and colder temperatures. Six of us left our camp at 0645hrs and made it to VK where we switched our military vehicles for a comfortable VW van. Before departing, we had to go over a lengthy checklist, and to no one's surprise, our vehicle was missing some important items, so we had to wait for all of this to be straightened out. We ended up leaving thirty minutes late, and Major Roy Hillier, the person I was supposed to meet with, just happened to be at the wrong place at the right time, so magically we arrived at our meeting place at the same time. I then spent the next five and a half hours running around the city with Roy and a team of about ten Americans who will be handling their team planning prior to the 1999 CISM Military World Games. The Americans sent twice as many people as Canada, and not one of them has any experience planning for a major sporting event. It is hard to believe that people can be this stupid.

At approximately 1400hrs the rain began mixing with snow, and I knew our return trip was destined to be challenging. After prying the nursing staff away from the PX where they had the irresistible opportunity to buy things at higher prices than they would pay in Canada, we began our journey home at 1540hrs. At this point in time, it was snowing heavily. Despite the snowfall, our drive was going very well until we got to a small road heading out of Karlovac. Here we encountered an oncoming transport truck with a piggybacked unit that suddenly began jackknifing out of control. We managed to avoid a collision, but when the dust settled, the front end of the truck was stuck in the ditch on the left, and the back end of the truck was stuck in the ditch on the right. The net result was a complete roadblock.

I knew immediately we were in for a loooooong night, and I wasn't disappointed. We had no option of backtracking and detouring around the accident site because the idiots that drive in this part of the world had decided to park in both lanes. We couldn't even take a side road around the accident because none had been proven to be mine-free. We also couldn't call anyone to let them know where we were because none of our civilian or issued phone cards would work. So, we sat there for three hours until the authorities managed to tow the transport truck out of the way. By the time we were finally able to move, the road was covered with a great deal of snow.

Moving at a snail's pace, we had to crawl through a five-and-a-half-kilometre-long bottleneck of backed-up traffic. Little did we know that the traffic jam obscured our exit road to VK, so we continued down the wrong road for an hour before realizing that nothing looked familiar. We stopped for directions and were told that VK was only thirty-two kilometres from where we were. What we weren't told was that this would be over increasingly narrow dirt roads in the mountains. At one point we had to put chains on the front tires because the van could not climb the hills without them. In the end, our two-hour trip from Zagreb to VK took nine hours, but on the positive side, we did get to see a whole lot of rural Croatia.

In VK, we swapped our van for an Iltis and an MLVW truck and made it back to camp by midnight. While the trip was a classic Menard disaster, my guardian angels ensured that we all returned safe and sound. I don't think I will embark on any more misadventures before I leave for Canada. Even if I wanted to go somewhere else, I doubt that I could find anyone desperate enough to travel with me.

———

28 January 1999

All of the snow that fell last night melted today, and Stalag Coralici is once again a veritable sea of slush.

I had the opportunity to meet Captain Edora's replacement this morning, and he seems like a very keen guy. The CAF sent him here despite the fact that he will be getting out in June '99, and they will be short an MO in Coralici for the final two months of the tour. Apparently, my replacement is aware of this and is willing to cover both jobs for the last two months of his deployment. This will be challenging because the last two months are usually fairly busy with handover preparations along with 380 medicals that have to be done. Best of luck.

At 1030 hours this morning, one of our HLVW wrecker trucks ran into a family driving a VW Golf. The wrecker was scratched in a few places, but the VW was totally decimated. There were four people in the VW: a two-year-old girl and her grandfather died on impact, and two others were seriously injured. Neither of our soldiers was physically injured, but they were badly shaken up by this horrible event. Our driver was given a breathalyzer test on the scene, and fortunately, the results confirmed he had no alcohol in his system. He also had a blood sample taken to determine if he was impaired by something other than alcohol. I am not certain if these guys were rookies or part of Roto 3. What is really scary is that the accident happened in the same town we were stuck in last night.

One of our soldiers was charged with being drunk this morning. He had a good tour, performed very well and was heading home in several days. So instead of doing the smart thing and waiting until he left the theatre to celebrate, he decided to consume more than his two-can limit last night. He was so drunk he urinated all over his bed and the floor of his sea container. When he got up this morning, he was still very intoxicated, and that's when the sparks began to fly. I am sure when all is said and done, he will end up with a large fine and an all-expense paid trip to the Crowbar Hotel. What a terrible way to end your deployment.

Both of today's incidents serve to illustrate why commanding officers worry so much when deployed operations start to wind down. As the time to head home rapidly approaches, soldiers commonly begin to relax, and this increases the chances of making mistakes or bad decisions. In both of these cases, I am sure the soldiers involved will never forget what happened to them today. Please Lord, help every-one who survived today's accident to heal quickly and to know that you love them. Amen.

———————

30 January 1999

Today there were two big events on the agenda: the transfer of authority for the Battle Group and the arrival of my replacement. I'll let you guess which event was of greater significance to me. We awoke to the coldest weather we have had to endure in well over a month, and once again the soldiers were expected to be on parade. Mercifully, the event was short and sweet, and in the end the CO of 3 RCR handed over the control of the AOR to the CO of 2 RCR. At the conclusion of this cer-emony, virtually the entire Battle Group headed off for Canada, and the few of us who remain find ourselves living in a sea of fresh new faces.

I was given my Personnel Evaluation Report (PER – essentially my deployment report card) today, and I doubt I will ever see a better evaluation even if I serve until I am one hundred years old. Unfortu-nately, without the ability to "parlez-vous le ding dong," I will almost certainly remain a lowly major.

This afternoon, the PsychO and I went up to VK to pick up our replacements, and they both looked pretty beat up after their long journey. To make matters worse, they of course had to go through the endless clearing-in process. LCol Ricard is my replacement, and this is his fifth tour and his third marriage – I wonder if these two statis-tics are somehow related. This is his second time in Bosnia, but he has never been the medical advisor and never been sentenced to do time in Stalag Coralici. In an effort to roll out the welcome carpet for this seasoned veteran, the contingent somehow managed to lose his entire luggage. We looked in every possible place that it could be, and eventually we found the luggage that our pharmacist had been missing for two weeks but not a single item that belonged to LCol Ricard. What a wonderful way to start your seven-month tour.

In preparation for the arrival of my replacement, I spent the morning packing up all my belongings and gave my sea container a thorough cleaning. I have decided to live my last few days in camp in my office rather than share a room with four other people. I have a cot, and I patched up some of the holes in the walls to try and make the place warm enough to safely sleep in. Looking at the pile of stuff that I have sitting in my office, I have no idea how I am ever going to get it all into the luggage that I have. I think I will pray that the Lord will pull off a kind of reverse of the loaves and the fishes miracle.

31 January 1999

It's my last Sunday in theatre, and I am ready to head home. The weather here remained rather cold today. The new camp CSM and I went for what would be my last opportunity to experience the pain of running the infamous club route with its eighteen-minute hill. I will miss the challenge that this run presented to me every weekend.

Father McDonald said his last Mass with us, as he will also be heading home. I will miss these intimate celebrations, but I am looking forward to worshipping the Lord with friends and family in our beautiful little church back in Russell.

The new crew was a little excited this morning because a local man drove up to the front gate, pulled out a shotgun and killed two dogs. Who could blame the gate guards for being upset by a stranger firing off a gun in their immediate vicinity, because it wasn't all that long ago that these people were killing each other. Welcome to the wonderful world of Bosnia, boys and girls.

LCol Ricard got to attend his first AOR briefing, and then we went over how to do the all-important EpiNATO statistics. I hope he has as much fun preparing these statistics as I did because they are, in my opinion, largely a waste of time. After that, we went for a tour of Stalag Coralici, and I pointed out the many highlights he will get to enjoy for the next seven months. After we examined the helicopter landing zone, I mentioned to him that during the handover period there have been hardly any choppers coming to visit us. No more than five minutes after I said this, a helicopter touched down in our camp. At the conclusion of my guided tour, I gave him a handover package that should answer just about any question he might have. Tomorrow we will see what questions he has, and then I will try to fade away into the background. The remaining Roto 3 staff members are also fading into the background as the rookies assume the reins of power. I find that we are becoming more and more like ghosts, as the world we find ourselves trapped in continues to move on. There appear to be very few people here who are even aware that we actually exist. It is definitely time to pass on the torch and head home.

February 1999

1 February 1999

One more beautiful morning run in the mountains and one less day in theatre. It is amazing to watch our camp rapidly change as the folks of Roto 4 attempt to put their own mark on everything. As I watch them, I am reminded of my own first month in theatre when I spent many an hour running around trying to scrounge up a few basic items to make my life in camp more comfortable. Based on experience, I have come to believe that it is only normal for people to rearrange a new workspace to establish some sense of ownership. Although my office is a model of workplace efficiency (not!), I am sure that even my successor can hardly wait for me to get on the happy bus and get the hell out of here so he can change everything around.

The new staff have had their first person with a chest pain come in for admission, and it was very reminiscent of our first few days in theatre when one of our soldiers came in with a heart attack that damaged the inferior wall of his heart. The soldier seen today appears to be doing fine, but he will still be admitted to the hospital for closer observation. I sincerely hope that the new medical staff encounter fewer serious medical problems than we did.

Janet and I have decided to spend our first night together in a nice hotel for two reasons: for privacy, and because I will be finished my clearing-in process very late at night, and we don't think it would be smart to drive all the way home on potentially slippery roads while we are both exhausted. As it turns out, Janet has rented the honeymoon suite, and I am not sure if her intentions are entirely platonic. I certainly hope not.

I have essentially completed my handover with LCol Ricard, and I wish there were some way I could get out of his hair, but this is difficult when I am still sleeping in the office that he recently inherited from me.

One of the medical assistants that I came to know and enjoy working with left me a note the night he left. Here is what he said: "Many men I have met on my path – strong, weak, wise and blind. Unfortunately, few decent men. Thanks for being one of the few." This simple note means a great deal to me because it expresses exactly how I feel about one of the greatest influences in my life – my father. Thank you, Lord, for blessing me with a great set of parents. Please continue to watch over them. Amen.

---

2 February 1999

It is getting late, and I will be leaving this camp forever at 0445hrs tomorrow morning. Sitting in an office that no longer belongs to me is a very odd feeling. It is with some real reluctance that I am relinquishing the responsibilities that I have been privileged to hold for these last seven months. A great deal of work goes into taking good care of ill and injured soldiers, and I believe that our medical team has met and exceeded that standard. This has been the best military experience of my career, and I have learned many lessons that I hope will hold me in good stead in the future. Probably the greatest blessing has been the opportunity to work with and get to know a whole bunch of wonderful soldiers, from the Contingent Commander on down. I have met the new Commander, and it seems as though he was carved from the same stone as Col Natynczyk. If this is true, then Roto 4 will surely have a successful tour of duty.

The ASC and the UMS staff are beginning to gel into a cohesive team. They will need this partnership to survive the next seven months of constant and potentially life-threatening demands that they will encounter. The new Medical Advisor is a very bright and experienced soldier. I am not sure how much clinical medicine he has practised in the last few years, but I hope that he is able to practise as much medicine as he feels comfortable with.

The bunch of us who are flying out tomorrow had to pack up and then load up all our accompanied baggage at 1300hrs. All that we have left is a small carry-on kit with very little in it. I even had to give up my Gerber multi-tool and Bear Jaws, and I must say that I do feel rather naked without them on my person.

Dear Lord, you have looked after us so far on this challenging journey, please remain by my side and get me and the other soldiers home safely to the arms of our loved ones. I ask this in the name of your son, Jesus Christ. Amen.

Good night, Stalag Coralici – as strange as this may sound, I will truly miss you!

---

3 February 1999

We got up at 0400hrs this morning to catch our happy bus out of town. It's funny how no one was complaining about leaving at this time of day. The bus took us to VK where we were put through what is referred to as a Departure Assistance Group (DAG). This took all of forty-five minutes, and then we waited another two and a half hours for our bus to head up to Zagreb.

Dr. Begovic was kind enough to meet me at the Zagreb airport, and I got to say farewell to this gentleman whom I have come to know and greatly respect. I certainly hope he and Aida survive all the changes that are coming to this part of the world.

Our airbus took off at 1300hrs, and as we were about to board, they asked everyone to check their boarding pass to see if they had a red slash through it. Anyone with a red slash was allocated a first-class seat and got to board the aircraft first. I sure don't know why they do these kinds of things because it only serves to piss off the troops.

We had an eleven-hour flight with a brief refuelling stop in Shannon, Ireland. I slept as much as I could because I wanted to be at least semi-conscious when I finally got to see Janet. After landing in Trenton at approximately 1830hrs, we had to collect all our luggage and clear customs. Although there were only 147 of us on the plane, this process managed to drag on for ninety minutes. During processing, I was informed that I was the senior military person on board, and as such, I would have to be the parade commander when we finally arrived in Petawawa. Never having done this before, I spent the next three and a half hours mentally rehearsing all my commands in the hope that I wouldn't cause myself too much embarrassment.

Once we cleared customs, we loaded all our equipment into the back of a trailer truck and headed out on our three-hour bus ride to Petawawa, where 147 families were patiently awaiting our return. When we finally arrived at our destination, I was quickly taken off the bus and given a review of what they expected me to do for the parade – it was very different from what I had just spent the last few hours rehearsing. In the meantime, everyone else was being held in a corridor and not allowed to see their families. Considering the circumstances, I felt it would be very disrespectful to prolong the separation of our troops from their families. So we quickly formed up into three ranks and marched into the building with a piper accompanying us. I consider the parade to have been a success for two reasons: I didn't end up being court-martialed, and no one died! When I dismissed the troops, they all ran off to the embrace of loving arms. It was nice to see Janet, and after another one and a half hours of processing, we were finally on the highway headed for the honeymoon suite at the luxurious Best Western. I couldn't think of a better way to end this adventure than to spend the evening with my best friend, my wife and the mother of my children. Thank you, Lord, for getting me home safe and sound, and thank you for watching over my loved ones while I was away.

---

4 February 1999

No words can describe how happy I was to wake up this morning in Canada, with my wife beside me and no weapon on my belt. My morning run was on snowmobile trails, and it felt unnatural not to be concerned about having my legs blown off by a land mine.

On our way home, we stopped by the Ottawa Civic Hospital to check up on our soldier with ulcerative colitis – my last official duty as a part of the Roto 3 medical team. It turns out that he was very ill when he finally landed in Canada, and he ended up having the diseased section of his large intestine surgically removed. The good news is that he is making a good recovery and should be back on his feet in the next few weeks. He did not expect someone from our medical team to take the time to come and see him, but I felt this was the right thing to do. Our visit meant a great deal to his wife, and she thanked me for helping to save her husband's life. I sincerely hope this young man heals well and that he can continue his service in the Canadian Armed Forces.

There was no welcome home parade when we finally reached Russell. It was just the same calm and peaceful place that I left behind to spend 209 days in a war-torn country. I hope the work that we did as part of Roto 3 helps the people of Bosnia rebuild a nation that was destroyed by many years of fighting.

As I mentioned at the beginning of this book, prior to being selected for this tour of duty, I was feeling burnt-out and was praying for a much-needed change in my life. God answered my prayer by sending me to Bosnia, and while I didn't understand this decision at the time, in retrospect it was the best thing that could have happened to me. I returned home re-energized, with my sense of humour restored and with a greater appreciation for all the blessings I have in my life. God truly does work in mysterious ways, and I will be forever grateful. Amen.

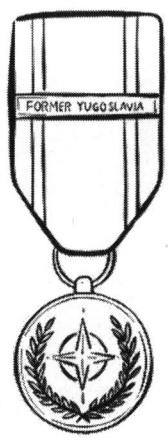

Final Note

The Canadian Contingent Stabilization Force (CCSFOR) that I was privileged to work with consisted of over thirteen hundred Canadian soldiers who worked tirelessly to provide a safe and stable environment so that other international agencies could work to help rebuild this completely shattered country. Ethnic tensions, land mines, mountainous terrain, bad weather and serpentine roads all served to make this a dangerous place to work.

In addition to helping to keep the peace, the Canadian Contingent was very engaged in terms of providing humanitarian aid. This type of aid involved a variety of initiatives including carrying out Operation Shoebox, providing medical and dental supplies to local hospitals and clinics, renovating the psychiatric facility in Bihac, purchasing and installing air conditioning units in the surgical rooms at the Bihac hospital, repairing schools, constructing bridges, providing children's winter clothing, providing health care personnel at local medical and dental clinics, assisting with surgeries at a local hospital, assessing children who were injured by the weapons of war, clearing land mines and other unexploded ordnances, and providing food to families in need. I sincerely hope that all this work helps the people of Bosnia to rebuild their country because it was very expensive – it cost hundreds of millions of dollars and the lives of eleven young soldiers.

Lord, I am very grateful for being allowed to return safe and sound to my family and would like to sign off by asking you to help the families of those soldiers who were not so fortunate. Amen. Menard out!

Where They Ended Up

Colonel Walter Natynczyk (Commander of CCSFOR Bosnia) – enjoyed an amazing career and retired as the Chief of Defence Staff.

Corporal Kim Holland (Queen of Operation Shoebox) – retired from the Canadian Forces shortly after her deployment to Bosnia. She moved back to Thessalon Ontario where she continues to work with her family in the building and hardware business. She served on the town council for eight years and is a proud member of a veteran's motorcycle group.

Major Sylvain Lavoie (one of the Three Amigos) – retired in 2009 as a Lieutenant Colonel and pursued a second career with NATO.

Captain Kerry Horlock – retired a Brigadier General.

LCol Mike Jorgenson (CO of the 3 RCR Battle Group) – survived a Hercules aircraft crash and eventually became the Director of Army Training. He retired as a Brigadier General.

Captain Peter Clifford – was inducted as an Officer in the Order of St. John. He served as the Deputy Surgeon General and retired as a Colonel.

Dr. Igor Begovich (the medical liaison to the Canadian contingent) – passed his American medical boards, did his specialty training in anesthesiology in the USA and now works in the USA as a cardiovascular anesthesiologist.

Jenny Tuls (the Camp's rubber doll) – is likely still tramping around Bosnia.

Me (the medical advisor to the Canadian Contingent) – inducted as an Officer in the Order of St. John, retired from the CAF, and continues to practice clinical sport medicine and serve as the Surgeon General's Specialist Advisor in Sport Medicine.

About the Author

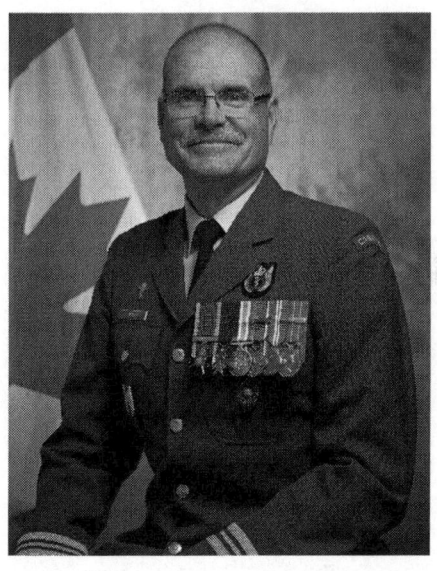

Major (Retired) D.C. Menard OMM, CD2, BPE, MA, MD, Dip. Sport Med

Major (Retired) Darrell Menard is Métis and served forty years in the CAF. He and wife, Janet, have raised three children: Nathan, Matthew and Rebecca. Darrell has an honours degree in physical education, a master's degree in exercise physiology, a Doctor of Medicine degree, and a CASEM (Canadian Academy of Sport and Exercise Medicine) Diploma in Sport Medicine.

Darrell has been a competitive runner since 1969 and won a gold medal with Jacques Pilon for the 1500 metre event in 1980, at what is now called the Paralympic Games. He also represented the Canadian Armed Forces at five World Military Cross-Country Championships. He has held the Canadian Armed Forces record for 1500 metres for forty-eight years. He has been a recreational curler for fourteen years and helps coach youth and adult curlers at the Russell Curling Club.

During his career, Darrell has worked at twenty-five major games, including as a member of the 1980 and 2016 Canadian Paralympic teams and the 2012 Canadian Olympic team. He continues to work as the Surgeon General's Specialist Advisor in Sport Medicine and as an adjunct professor in the University of Ottawa School of Nursing. He is also the author of the CASEM's Ask the Expert article series, and has his own sport medicine practice in Russell, Ontario.

Darrell has been named an Officer of the Order of Military Merit and an Officer of the CISM Order of Merit. He has also been inducted into the Canadian Armed Forces Sports Hall of Fame, and the University of Alberta's Sports Wall of Fame.

Manufactured by Amazon.ca
Bolton, ON